ADVANCE PRAISE FOR

EFFORTLESS HEALING

"*Effortless Healing* will cause a simple revolution in your health. I have been a fan of Dr. Mercola's work for many years, and this book is the synthesis of his wisdom; it will help anyone feel better quickly."

—DANIEL G. AMEN, M.D., author of *Change Your Brain, Change Your Life* and coauthor of *The Daniel Plan*

"Dr. Mercola has been one of the leading teachers of health for a quarter century, and with this book he has done an admirable job of succinctly summarizing and making accessible to all decades of accumulated knowledge. Those fortunate enough to read it will likely be rewarded with many extra years of health and life."

—RON ROSEDALE, M.D., founder of DrRosedale.com

"If you want to improve your health, embrace the simple but elegant recommendations of Dr. Mercola. He is consistently ahead of the rest of the medical community, and his approach is solid and based on state-of-the-art scientific evidence."

—RICHARD JOHNSON, M.D., professor of medicine, University of Colorado, and author of *The Fat Switch*

"*Effortless Healing* is a very worthwhile read not only for the public but also for health care practitioners, who need to be teaching their patients the importance of following the advice in this book. These pages contain foundational truths that are well-researched and have already been proven effective in patients by Dr. Mercola, by me, and by other practitioners. If people, especially those in the United States, would act upon the simple, doable recommendations in this book, I predict that the incidence of obesity and most chronic diseases would drop dramatically. Read *Effortless Healing* and then apply its wisdom in your life so that you also can experience vitality and longevity!"

—W. LEE COWDEN, M.D., M.D.(H.), chairman of the Scientific Advisory Board, Academy of Comprehensive Integrative Medicine

"Dr. Mercola is a national, and indeed international, leader in the natural health and organic movements. His new book, *Effortless Healing,* is essential reading for all health conscious and concerned Americans, giving us the information and inspiration we need to heal ourselves and revitalize public health."

—RONNIE CUMMINS, founder and director,
Organic Consumers Association

"A true visionary who champions freedom of thought, Dr. Mercola has empowered millions of people around the world to take control of their health with commonsense advice. He makes it easy to understand why healing and staying well is something everyone can do safely, effectively, and naturally by simply making more conscious choices."

—BARBARA LOE FISHER, cofounder and president,
National Vaccine Information Center

"Dr. Mercola's latest book, *Effortless Healing,* will greatly expand the general public's awareness about some of the latest concepts and challenges facing our food choices and our health. He shares one bit of valuable medical information after another and then expands it, and discusses how these suggestions can be more readily implemented and effortlessly expanded to improve the health of all Americans."

—DORIS J. RAPP, M.D., environmental medical
specialist and pediatric allergist

"In his latest book, *Effortless Healing,* the father of modern nutrition provides a hands-on, easy-to-implement, and yes, effortless guide that empowers you to overcome disease and take charge of your health. Whether you want to lose fat fast, turn back the clock, or simply eat more vegetables, this book provides a comprehensive arsenal of tools to reach your goals, maintain optimal health, and become your very best self."

—JJ VIRGIN, *New York Times* bestselling author
of *The Virgin Diet* and *Sugar Impact Diet*

EFFORTLESS HEALING

9 Simple Ways to
Sidestep Illness, Shed Excess Weight,
and Help Your Body Fix Itself

DR. JOSEPH MERCOLA

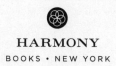

HARMONY
BOOKS · NEW YORK

Published in the United States by Harmony Books, an imprint of the Crown Publishing Group, a division of Penguin Random House LLC, New York.
crownpublishing.com

Harmony Books is a registered trademark, and the Circle colophon is a trademark of Penguin Random House LLC.

Originally published in hardcover in the United States by Harmony Books, an imprint of the Crown Publishing Group, a division of Penguin Random House LLC, New York, in 2015.

Some of the content in this work has been adapted from material appearing on Dr. Mercola's successful website, Mercola.com.

Library of Congress Cataloging-in-Publication Data
Mercola, Joseph.
Effortless healing : 9 simple ways to sidestep illness,
shed excess weight, and help your body fix itself /
Dr. Joseph Mercola.
1. Nutrition. 2. Diet. 3. Health behavior.
4. Self-care, Health. I. Title.
RA784.M47 2015
613.2—dc 3 2014022046

ISBN 978-1-101-90289-9
eBook ISBN 978-0-553-41798-2

Printed in the United States of America

Cover design by Nicole Caputo
Cover photograph by ClaudioVentrella/iStock
Author photograph: Courtesy of Mercola.com

10 9 8 7 6 5 4 3 2 1

First Paperback Edition

I would like to dedicate this book to
my Health Liberty partners.
I am lucky to know such brilliant and caring people.
Thank you, Barbara Loe Fisher, Ronnie Cummins,
Paul Connett, and Charlie Brown.
You have sacrificed so much to prevent the needless pain
and suffering that occurs in this world and inspire hope
that we can advance our global health consciousness.

Contents

FOREWORD

Y ou have been given a nearly flawless gift that's been in the making for over two million years. Your DNA, your code of life, has been refined and polished over countless generations to provide you with optimal health, functionality, and longevity.

And yet, in the last one half of one percent of our time as humans, we as a species are experiencing a dramatic challenge to our ability to stave off disease.

The explosive increase in the prevalence of diabetes, obesity, hypertension, Alzheimer's disease, and other degenerative conditions is not a manifestation of any sudden change in our genetics. Indeed, genetics researchers would be hard pressed to identify any significant changes in the human genome compared with that of humans from 20,000 years ago.

So what has changed? If the genetic blueprint that codes for health and longevity has remained constant, what are the factors that have been introduced that have corrupted the message from this seemingly immutable code?

As it turns out, the notion that our DNA represents a fixed and immutable code is now looked upon as antiquated science. What we've come to understand is that our genetic code is actually aggressively dynamic in its expression. The very genes that were viewed as being locked in a glass case are now seen as responding moment to moment to any number of environmental influences.

This, the science of *epigenetics*, opens up not only a new way of conceptualizing the behavior of our genes but also, more important, provides a new perspective for the understanding of the rampant health issues that characterize the modern Western world.

Epigenetic research reveals that our lifestyle choices—the foods we eat, the supplements we take, the exercise we pursue, and even the emotional content of our daily experiences—are all involved in orchestrating chemical reactions that activate or deactivate parts of our genome that will either code for outcomes that threaten health and pave the way for disease or create an internal environment conducive to longevity and disease resistance.

That is the gift of this new understanding of genes and their expression. The profound upside of this new paradigm is that it reveals that each of us has the opportunity to modify our own genetic expression and change our health destiny.

In the pages that follow, Dr. Mercola will empower you with the ability to rewrite your story as it relates to your future health. By paying close attention to the information he presents, you will learn how you can positively influence the expression of your own DNA to improve and preserve your health and extend your life.

And whether it's shifting your diet to one that welcomes fat back to the table, enjoying more sunshine, dedicating yourself to getting more sleep, or even making a point to go barefoot from time to time, each of the empowering recommendations in *Effortless Healing* is designed to reestablish life-sustaining and life-enhancing communication with your most precious gift, your code of life.

DAVID PERLMUTTER, M.D.

EFFORTLESS HEALING

Introduction

You may think that I have always been dedicated to health, but that is absolutely not the case. I was raised on dessert after most meals, doughnuts, Twinkies, chips, and ice cream. In other words, I grew up eating the typical American diet. My parents did the best that they could in trying to provide us with home-cooked meals. But they didn't know then what we know now about nutrition. As a result, by the time I was in high school, nearly half of my teeth had cavities and my face and back were riddled with acne. I was clearly, like so many others are today, working against my body, not with it.

It's a funny beginning for someone who would end up as one of the world's leading advocates for using food as medicine. Yet my experiences fueled me to help the average person—who is used to eating whatever tastes good and is struggling with chronic conditions, yet never connected these two dots.

Over the last three decades, I have treated more than 25,000 patients as a physician, diligently reviewed a huge array of nutritional approaches, written two *New York Times* bestselling books, and built the most visited natural health website in the world that is dedicated to educating readers about proven ways to improve their health; Mercola.com now reaches 25 million readers every month.

The trait that is most responsible for my journey to being a champion of high-quality nutrition is my love of reading. It was an article in *Parade* magazine in 1968 that started me on my current path. The article was about Dr. Ken Cooper and his brand-new book, *Aerobics*. At that point in time, hardly anyone exercised regularly. (When I went jogging back then on the West Side of Chicago, people would throw rocks and cans at me, because they assumed I was a criminal running from the scene of a crime.) I read his book and started on a now nearly fifty-year-long commitment to fitness. Of course, my views have evolved over time. I'm no longer a slavish devotee to what we now call cardio—in fact, I'm just the opposite. But more on that later in the book.

Back then, practicing medicine wasn't even on my radar. I entered college with an engineering major and changed to premed only after I started. I was very traditional in my approach to medicine in those early days: for six years before medical school, I worked as a pharmacist's apprentice. I enjoyed the job and felt the drugs I helped dispense were a beneficial solution to our patients' health care challenges.

That indoctrination continued through medical school, even though the difference between the medical mainstream and me was already starting to surface: my fellow students nicknamed me Dr. Fiber for my dedication to fiber and its relation to gut health. (My understanding of the true drivers of gut health has continued to evolve over many years of study and research—more on that in Healing Principle 6.)

As a family practitioner, I was a paid speaker for the drug companies and would fly around the country on their dime, hailing the benefits of estrogen replacement therapy.

In the early years of my private practice, my focus was

treating depression, because it was such an underdiagnosed dilemma. People were clearly suffering, but the only treatment I knew of was drugs. Thousands of my patients received hope for healing in the form of a prescription I'd written for them. I didn't know better at the time.

So how did I make the transition to natural medicine?

In the mid-1980s I read a book called *The Yeast Connection* by William Crook, M.D. It described people making miraculous recoveries from treating yeast overgrowth. I recognized the symptoms he described in many of my patients. At this point, I ignored Crook's dietary recommendations and instead used the antifungal drugs he recommended for treatment, and, of course, that failed miserably. But in the early 1990s, I read the book again. By then I had gained some wisdom, so this time I took his dietary recommendations to heart. They worked incredibly well and opened my eyes to the power of food—not drugs—as medicine. As I began attending health conferences, I realized that there was a wide network of physicians using natural therapies to treat their patients.

As I applied these new skills to my practice, I was thrilled to see so many people getting much better using diet and lifestyle modifications. I was so convinced by these outcomes that I decided to change my practice to natural medicine and refused to see patients who were unwilling to embark on a journey to address the foundational causes of their illness.

This was a serious risk to my income, as I was a solo practitioner, and I wound up losing 75 percent of my patients. But like most decisions in life that are made for the right reason, this one worked out really well, and my practice was soon filled by all the referrals I was getting from successfully treated patients. I eventually started seeing patients from all over the world.

It was quite a shift in my view of myself—from the healer who could administer the drugs that would "fix" a patient's health, to more of an educator who could help people learn how to cultivate the power to heal. Your body was designed to be healthy without requiring a drug. Give it what it needs to thrive, and it will typically regenerate itself without any outside interventions. This innate restorative tendency is what I call "Effortless Healing."

That shift—to empowering people to become their own healers—became the driving force of my medical practice. Coupled with my passion for research and separating the spin from the truth, that desire led me to be an early force of change in many areas of health that are now commonplace: the GMO labeling debate, the phasing out of "silver" mercury fillings worldwide, ending fluoridation of municipal water supplies, the importance of vitamin D as it relates to optimal health and cancer prevention, and the importance of omega-3 fats like krill oil.

Another passion of mine has always been technology—I took my first computer programming class in 1969. One piece of being a family doctor that frustrated me was having patients come in asking for a drug or a treatment they had seen on TV. As a professional who worked eighty hours a week or more, I rarely had the time or interest to watch TV. I spent every free moment reviewing the literature that was now freely available on the Internet.

In 1997, I started Mercola.com as a place to chronicle my evolution as a physician while I learned and implemented more and more about natural medicine. I decided to share everything I learned at the many dozens of weekend courses I would take as well. I would hold nothing back and share everything with the reader as if he or she were a patient seeing me in my office. It was all free advice.

My aim for Mercola.com has always been to provide my unadulterated views and to share my passion for finding the best researchers and bringing their work to a wider audience. I have never accepted ads or sponsors, as that could lead to potential conflicts of interest. And for the first four years of the site's life, I sold no products. The only reason I started selling them was that by that time, I had spent $500,000 in developing and maintaining the site, and the bills were only increasing.

It was clear that this model would not scale well. So we now sell products that I or my family use and that are of the highest quality. Doing this supplies the funds to support my mission: to bring readers the best information available so that they can optimize their health.

About four years ago I modified my goal from simply educating the public to affecting global change in health policy and industry practices. I started the Health Liberty Initiative so I could take a leadership role and work directly on catalyzing change in the food and medical industries.

This initiative was necessary to bring together diverse groups, whose intentions were aligned but strategies were not. My hope for the Health Liberty Initiative is to raise our collective level of consciousness as it relates to food, health, and our environment. Many people don't realize that the USDA, which is designed to ensure the safety and quality of our food supply, sets our nation's agriculture policy as well as our dietary standards— a classic example of the fox guarding the henhouse.

One of the reasons Mercola.com is so popular is because my experience treating so many patients has helped me to translate complex medical jargon into easy-to-understand, everyday language and turn hard-to-understand studies into easily actionable advice. This book is my effort to compile the best of the information shared over the last two decades and put it into an inspiring guide that will help you avoid the many pitfalls of the conventional approach to health. Rather than rely on expensive and potentially dangerous drugs, I will help you understand how you can effortlessly modify your diet to achieve your health goals.

In this book, I will guide you through the nine principles of healing, which will help you choose more skillfully what and when to eat, what to drink, how and when to be physically active, and how to incorporate more exposure to nature into your life while also protecting yourself from the toxins that are increasingly present in the environment. You will also learn how to achieve the new health goals you make as a result of reading this book.

My mission in writing this book is the same as my mission in creating the website and running the Health Liberty Initiative, and it will never change: to inform you of the details that are frequently omitted from the often manipulated health stories you hear or read about in the media; and to help you remove the roadblocks to wellness—such as subpar food and contaminated beverages—so that your body can do what it was designed to do effortlessly: stay well.

It is also to preserve your freedom of choice when it comes to how you manage your health. Whether the subject is medication, the food you eat, the water you drink, or the seeds you grow, I believe you deserve the right to choose what goes into your body. And you deserve to be told the truth about the health consequences of your decisions.

You hold in your hands the power to be healthy, and I am honored to be part of your effortless journey to claiming and exercising that power.

Part One

Effortless Health

Chapter 1

What Effortless Healing Is, and Why You Need It

If you have opened this book because you are challenged with a chronic health condition, excess weight, or a general malaise, I'm not surprised. Statistically speaking, you are much more likely to be some level of sick than you are to be well.

You might question how we could still be so far from understanding health and curing diseases. After all, the forty years we've spent fighting the War on Cancer has resulted in $500 billion in expenditures, yet the death rate has changed little.[1] Medical science in general could be implicated: cancer researcher Glenn Begley attempted to replicate fifty-three "landmark studies"— conducted by top labs and published in major medical journals— and could only reproduce six.[2] That's an 89 percent failure rate.

Obesity rates are at an all-time high and rising—the Gallup-Healthways Well-Being poll, which has been monitoring body mass index (BMI) since 2008, found that in 2013 the number of obese Americans rose a full percentage point, after being basically flat for five years.[3] For the first time in human history, this generation will live a shorter time than their parents[4]—and this is despite spending an estimated $2.9 trillion in 2013 on health care in the U.S. alone.[5] How is that for progress?

The US Centers for Disease Control and Prevention (CDC) estimates that by 2050, one in three U.S. adults will have diabetes.[6] One in eight people aged sixty-five and over currently has Alzheimer's,[7] and that number is expected to rise to one in four within the next twenty years.

In its 2014 *World Cancer Report,* the World Health Organization reported a looming "human disaster" in the rising cancer rates—from 14 million new diagnoses reported in 2012 to an estimated 22 million annual diagnoses twenty years from now[8]— an increase of 57 percent. That means within two decades, 13 million people will die from cancer each year.

Asthma, hay fever, eczema, food allergies, lupus, multiple sclerosis, and other autoimmune diseases are all on the rise. According to some estimates, allergies and diseases of the immune system have doubled, tripled, or even quadrupled in the last few decades, with some studies indicating that more than half of the U.S. population has at least one clinically diagnosable allergy.[9] At an alarming rate, some people's immune systems are overreacting to substances that should be harmless, leading to allergies; others' immune systems are malfunctioning and attacking parts of their own body—the very definition of autoimmune disease.

If you seek relief from any of these conditions from your doctor, you are likely to leave his office with at least one prescription—and more likely, multiple—for pharmaceuticals. You may be shocked to learn that nearly 70 percent of all Americans are taking at least one prescription drug for a chronic or other medical condition, with antibiotics, antidepressants, and opioids topping the list.[10]

One in four senior citizens takes ten to nineteen pills a day.[11] But over the course of a year, the average adult age eighteen to sixty-five years old in the United States fills about a dozen prescriptions—unless they are over sixty-five, and then that number goes up to more than thirty a year.[12] In the pediatric population, one out of every five children takes at least one prescription drug every month, about 10 percent of them use two or more, and 1 percent use five or more drugs per month.[13]

These statistics, which are the latest available but still five to ten years old, are disturbing enough. But what is most shocking is that an average senior citizen who has been diagnosed with just five chronic conditions (osteoporosis, osteoarthritis, type 2 diabetes, hypertension, and COPD) will be taking a *minimum* of twelve different drugs *every day,* just to "treat" these conditions.[14]

If you consider that someone on hypertension drugs is most likely also to be on a statin to reduce cholesterol, this would bring it to thirteen prescription drugs taken every day. But if you add in drugs prescribed for other chronic conditions commonly associated with old age, such as GERD, angina, depression/mental illness, insomnia, sleep apnea, hot flashes, kidney disease, rheumatoid arthritis, and congestive heart failure,[15] that person could easily be taking as many as *two dozen or more* drugs a day! Since statistics show that three out of four older Americans have multiple chronic health conditions,[16] these numbers are not unrealistic.

But these "cures" come at a high cost—their side effects and even life-threatening adverse reactions can have a seriously detrimental impact on your health. After all, adverse reactions to prescription drugs were responsible for more than 2.3 million emergency room visits in the United States in 2011, up 84 percent from 1.3 million visits in 2005.[17] The FDA, an agency that doesn't protect us as it should, nonetheless cites that over 98,000 people died from adverse drug reactions in 2011—the sixth most common cause of death in 2011, according to the CDC.[18] There were over 573,000 incidents of adverse drug reactions with "serious" consequences—defined as hospitalization, life-threatening complications, disability, or other harmful outcomes.[19]

If you find yourself in the hospital, look out. Studies from the Institute of Medicine in 1999 showed that at least 44,000 people—and possibly as many as 98,000—die every year as a result of medical errors made in hospitals.[20] Ten years later, the Office of the Inspector General increased that number to 180,000 every year in Medicare patients alone.[21] And in 2013 a study in the *Journal of Patient Safety* suggested that the number could actually be as high as 440,000.[22] With so many dying just from the drugs they're using to "heal" every year, there's a good chance you personally know someone who suffered this unfortunate and unnecessary fate.

It's clear from these trends and the data that an ounce of prevention truly is worth a pound of cure. My intention in sharing the simple strategies within this book is to keep you and your family out of harm's way, so these mistakes never happen to you.

The Odds Are Stacked Against You

It is difficult to get a man to understand something when his salary depends upon not understanding it!
—Upton Sinclair

Why has it become so dangerous to seek help from the medical industry?

The best place to start is by looking at that nearly $3 trillion number I wrote about earlier. Pharmaceutical companies view your symptoms and see dollar signs. They spend billions every year advertising to you on TV and magazines to help their drugs find their way into your body.

There's the $5 billion they spend on direct-to-consumer marketing, of course. You've seen the ads showing silver-haired men grabbing their spouses with a knowing look in their eye, or the woman with a little black rain cloud over her head (a symbol of depression) that magically transforms into a rainbow after she takes a pill. Their oversimplified presentations—complete with long lists of side effects—have people feeling they know all there is to know about a drug, so they march in to their doctors' offices expecting a prescription. Even with the threat of numerous possible side effects, the lure of being able to simply take a pill and have a troublesome symptom magically "disappear" is just too alluring for many people to resist.

But if you don't buy what they're selling in their commercials, they spend another $16 billion every year to market to physicians so they'll use drugs as a primary solution to most of the health problems people have. Many people are completely unaware of the many ways in which they are being manipulated into taking dangerous and oftentimes completely unnecessary drugs.

Time to Lift the Veil . . .

Exposing pharmaceutical dangers can be quite hazardous in and of itself, as documents uncovered during a class-action lawsuit filed against Merck revealed disturbing plans to neutralize, destroy, and discredit doctors who warned about the dangers of Vioxx.

As reported on CBSNews.com, one e-mail from a Merck executive said about a doctor who disliked prescribing Vioxx: *"We may need to seek them out and destroy them where they live. . . ."*

It's quite clear that both doctors and the public at large are being manipulated for the sake of corporate profits. The pharmaceutical industry is not really in the business of promoting health; instead it makes money off disease. And when one market begins to dwindle, it simply creates a new one, by inventing yet another disease, usually by "upgrading" a common symptom to disease status. Need convincing? Keep reading. As CNN reported, in order to market its antidepressant Paxil, GlaxoSmithKline hired a PR firm to create a "public awareness campaign" about an "underdiagnosed" disease.

The disease? Social anxiety disorder . . . previously known as shyness.

You may have seen this campaign firsthand; ads stating "Imagine being allergic to people" were distributed widely, celebrities gave interviews to the press, and psychiatrists gave lectures on this new disease in the top twenty-five media markets. As a result, mentions of social anxiety in the press *rose from about 50 to more than 1 billion in just two years.* Social anxiety disorder became the "third most common mental illness" in the United States, and Paxil skyrocketed to the top of the charts as one of the most profitable and most prescribed drugs here. And that's just one example among so very many, including the pushes to sell drugs that treat high cholesterol (statin drugs such as Lipitor and Crestor) and acid reflux—two conditions that are much more effectively treated with simple dietary changes.

Physicians, sometimes unwittingly, also play a major role in the massive pharmaceutical deception perpetrated on the public, but their manipulations are often more obscure. Drug reps often give "gifts" to persuade doctors to prescribe the medications that they represent. These drug reps usually have no medical or scientific education. Instead, they're armed with some incredibly potent persuasion techniques.

Although the medical industry has established rules that limit face-to-face interactions between drug reps and doctors, drug companies influence doctor choices in numerous other ways, including sponsoring medical conferences and sponsoring third-party websites intended to provide "nondenominational" information about new drugs.[23] The method of indoctrination most difficult to detect is the "education" that doctors give to other doctors. A pharmaceutical company will pay individual doctors large fees to "educate" their colleagues about the benefits of a particular drug. Here, it's very easy for the doctor receiving the material to forget that the doctor presenting it is working on the drug company's behalf and not as an independent, well-educated, appropriate source of objective information.

As I mentioned in the introduction, I was one of their paid shills in the mid-1980s and so have firsthand experience on how it works. The company would pay my travel expenses and give me checks for as much as $5,000 for speaking. That may not seem like much to some people now, but thirty years ago for someone just graduating school with loads of debt, it was a major sum. It is a magnificent system, too, as you may feel that you are doing good and being paid to share your hard-earned knowledge, when the reality is that you are merely feeding the researchers' studies bought and paid for by the drug companies so they can sell more drugs.

And then there's the insidious drug industry–sponsored "education" that takes place in medical schools across the United States. For example, out of Harvard's 8,900 professors and lecturers, 1,600 admit that they or a family member have ties to drug companies that could bias their teaching or research.[24] In one year alone, the pharmaceutical industry contributed more than $11.5 million to Harvard for "research and continuing education classes."[25]

This goes on in virtually every medical institution in the United States and is a massively effective way to indoctrinate budding physicians. By influencing the recognized thought leaders of medicine, drug companies can outrageously influence the entire profession—this, combined with the previously discussed marketing efforts, and their political lobbying to change the laws to their advantage. As a patient, you don't have to fall victim to these tactics. You can learn to see right through the propaganda and stop being deceived by drug company lies and deceptions.

Chances are your doctor, even if he or she has good intentions and a desire to heal, not harm, has fallen prey to pharmaceutical marketing tactics. Most doctors simply do not have the time to re-search each drug, and they rely heavily on information from their pharmaceutical reps and from other "experts," that is, doctors who are receiving significant fees to talk about drug treatments.

One of my main goals in sharing this information is to keep you out of the doctor's office for anything other than preventive screenings and out of the hospital for anything but acute trau-mas. (Our medical system can be spectacularly effective in these instances.)

You absolutely *can* take control of your health. It doesn't have to be in anyone's hands but your own.

How Did We Get So Sick in the First Place?

The twenty-first century has brought about tremendous progress in technology, transforming culture, the way we communicate, and even the way we think. It's an exciting, paradigm-shifting time in history. But it's also a time fraught with lurking dangers.

Developments in technology have impacted our food supply, introducing genetically modified crops, processed foods that offer little or no nutritive value, pesticide-laden fruits and vegetables, and an overreliance on a handful of crops due to government farming policies. On top of these factors, today much of our food is pasteurized, irradiated, fumigated, and sterilized to the point that bacteria—even the good kind, which we rely on for our very existence (more on this in Healing Principle 6)—can no longer survive.

Ironically, the very advances that represent all that is modern in the world—hand sanitizers, treated water, factory farming—have created their own set of diseases. For example, triclo-san—an antibacterial chemical used in many soaps and hand sanitizers—has been shown to kill human cells,[26] and even the FDA admits it acts as an endocrine disruptor in animals.[27] When combined with chlorinated water, it produces chloroform[28]—a probable carcinogen according to the EPA.[29]

Scientists are now connecting the sudden increase in neurological disorders and autoimmune disease, and the steadily inclining rates of obesity, with these changes to our food supply and the greater changes in our environment. Although plenty of research is being done searching for "cures," a pernicious force is working just as hard to perpetuate the very conditions that are making so many people ill: greed.

If It Were Poison, It Wouldn't Be in the Grocery Store

I'm fond of exposing how much the drug, chemical, and junk food industries spend to manipulate and distort our perceptions. While the drug companies spend more than $21 billion a year, the food industry is spending *twice* that much to persuade you and your kids to choose highly processed convenience foods that will accelerate a massive decline in your health (and facilitate your need to use drugs to control your symptoms).

A whopping 90 percent of the foods that Americans purchase every year are processed foods. In a typical recent year, 2,800 new candies, desserts, ice creams, and snacks were introduced to the marketplace, compared with just 230 new fruits or vegetable products.

Food marketers do a masterful job at making fast foods and junk foods seem like a wise choice. They're relatively inexpensive, they taste good, and they make fixing dinner a snap. No longer do you need to fuss with actually cleaning or chopping a vegetable. Simply pop their prepared boxes of food into the microwave, and you're ready to go. (Frozen vegetables are the one exception, as they can be a healthful option if your choices of local vegetables are limited due to weather or geography.)

What the food industry neglects to tell you is that you will pay a heavy price for consuming a terrible diet. The overconsumption of these fake, overly processed foods is one of the major causes of a slew of chronic diseases facing the United States.

Why do they make these foods if they are so terrible?

One particular event in 1999 is an especially potent piece of the answer. As chronicled in an article in the *New York Times*,[30] in Minneapolis on April 8, 1999, the CEOs of eleven major food companies, including Nestlé, Kraft, Nabisco, General Mills, Coca-Cola, Mars, and Procter & Gamble, gathered at Pillsbury's headquarters to discuss the obesity epidemic. Many who attended weren't there to talk about how to end the obesity epidemic; rather, they were there to discuss how to defend themselves against claims that they were responsible in large part for creating it. At the time, Kraft was a subsidiary of Philip Morris, and their awareness of the role they played was thoroughly and smartly discussed in Michael Moss's *Salt, Sugar, Fat*: "As Philip Morris came under pressure for nicotine and cigarettes, it eventually started looking at the food divisions in light of the emerging obesity crisis. And there were moments in these internal documents where Philip Morris officials were saying to the food division, 'You guys are going to face a problem with salt, sugar, fat in terms of obesity of the same magnitude, if not more than [what] we're facing with nicotine right now. And you've got to start thinking about this issue and how you're going to deal with that.'"[31]

Yet still, most processed foods remain loaded with sugar, which has been shown to have devastating effects on overall health in the form of insulin resistance (which is a precursor to nearly every chronic disease; more on this in Healing

Principle 3), increased markers of heart disease such as triglycerides and the harmful form of cholesterol, and the development
of fat in and around the abdominal organs, which is also a major
predictor of chronic disease.[32]

High levels of sugar consumption are also linked with obesity,[33] diabetes,[34] and cancer.[35] Even worse, these harmful foods
are designed to be so tasty that they short-circuit your normal
feelings of satiety, making you crave more and more of them.
In fact, sugary processed foods have been shown to trigger the
same pathways in the brain associated with drug addiction.[36]
One study found that rats, when given the choice between a
sugary solution and cocaine, preferred the sugary solution—even
rats with a history of drug use.[37] For the sake of convenience
or good taste now, you are trading the most valuable asset you
have: your health.

If you read mainstream media, you may be convinced that all
you need to do is switch from one processed food to another—
from regular cookies to low-fat cookies, or from white bread to
whole wheat bread. I hate to burst this bubble, because I know
how alluring it is. But healing is not going to come from a box,
can, or bag. The companies that manufacture the foods that
come in those containers are interested in one thing only: selling
more of the foods they produce, and they will go to great lengths
to keep their bottom lines healthy. At some point in the future,
the junk food industry will likely find itself in a similar position
to the tobacco industry, acknowledging their role in the long-term
consequences of the health of millions of people.

The Way Out: Effortless Healing

You have the power to not only stop disease but also to har-
ness technology for your own and your family's good. All you

need is information, much of which is contained in these pages. Your body is equipped with powerful healing mechanisms that will typically self-correct most health problems, if you provide it with the nutrients it was designed for and requires. That's what I mean by Effortless Healing: getting out of your body's way and letting it naturally do what it's meant to do.

Your body was designed to be healthy. If you believe the media, you would think you were just a disaster waiting to happen and in need of the magical prescription from your doctor. However, nothing could be further from the truth. If you supply your body with an optimal diet and avoid exposure to the ever-increasing threats of toxins, then your body, following its design, will move toward health and away from disease without any conscious effort.

Your body is typically on autopilot to self-heal. For example, when you fall down and bruise yourself, aside from making sure you clean any open wounds to prevent any infections, you don't need to do anything more to get better. Your body has built-in repair systems to take care of the damage.

In this book, my goal is to help you tailor the latest and best health information to your unique self and circumstances. I'll guide you on how to track your physiological barometers of health. I'll also continuously remind you to check each change you make against how you feel as well as the results you experience. Because when it comes to creating regenerative health, there simply is no one-size-fits-all approach.

How hard is it to follow the advice in this book?

Some of the steps I counsel truly are effortless—letting the sun warm your skin, or kicking off your shoes when you're outside, for example. And some do require a little more effort or discipline at first—like, for example, weaning yourself from sugar.

But to advance from illness, pain, disease, and death to health, vitality, fitness, and happiness in your body and mind is a rewarding decision. And as soon as your body experiences the benefits of these choices, you will feel so much more invigorated that it will feel truly effortless to keep going.

Effortless Healing Is *Not* About Self-Deprivation

M any people feel that if they can't eat their favorite junk foods, they are being deprived. In reality, the sooner you change your eating habits, the sooner you'll enjoy increased energy, normalized weight, a better mood, and improved health overall. You are definitely trading up—the only thing you're denying yourself is feeling miserable.

Subsisting on junk foods alone is a surefire way to accelerate your aging process and compromise your health. There is just no way around it—if you want to reap a healthy life, you, a spouse, a relative, or someone you pay needs to invest some time in the kitchen and hopefully in the garden in preparing your food. Not only will you enjoy the health benefits, but the satisfaction of growing food, preparing meals, and being in control over what you put into your body can be a great feeling.

Following the Healing Principles in this book may require a little more time and energy than automatically reaching for a ready-made processed dish, but being healthy is not the difficult slog that so many think it is, especially when you give your body what it needs to thrive. Armed with the knowledge I've spent decades accumulating and am now sharing, you can:

- Add years to your lifespan
- Gain more energy than you know what to do with

And it can help you avoid:

- Cancer
- Heart disease
- Diabetes
- Arthritis
- Alzheimer's

Taking control of your food choices is a powerful way to activate Effortless Healing. There are others, which you'll learn about as well.

Your body has an innate desire to feel better, to be able to do and enjoy more. When you honor that desire by preparing your own food, gathering your own information, and making your own choices about what is truly healthy for your individual body, it will reward you with the support you need to keep going. Let this internal desire for health help you drop whatever mental resistance you may have to changing your daily routines. Let it help you make a transformative journey that feels so good, it becomes effortless.

Chapter 2

Before You Begin

Because you picked up this book, I'm guessing you are feeling more than ready to get started on your journey to Effortless Healing. There are just a few things to keep in mind and to do before you dive in.

First, I've presented the healing principles in order of importance. Each principle builds on the one before, so start with Healing Principle 1, "Drink Pure Water." Once you've upgraded your hydration, move on to Healing Principle 2. You're not running a race—you're embracing a lifestyle and seeking to improve it for the rest of your life, a lifestyle that will enable your body to do its job with the least effort on its—and your—part. As you systematically improve the food and nutrients you consume, you'll feel better and gain more and more energy to keep you motivated as you embrace each new principle.

Keeping Perspective Is Crucial

As you know, the conventional path to health and nutrition is associated with serious costs, both to your health and to your wallet. While embracing these Healing Principles is vital to your health, you've got to approach it with a light heart.

How you go about incorporating the principles will make a difference in how effective they will be for you. Your mental state is a vital component of your health, and feeling overwhelmed and stressed won't promote health—in fact, just the opposite, even if what's overwhelming you and stressing you out is making healthy changes.

So approach the changes I've outlined in this book with a sense of adventure, curiosity, and experimentation. Keep your mind focused on the positive changes you want, and not on the negative outcomes you're trying to avoid. In moments of doubt, ask yourself, would I like to regenerate or degenerate?

Honestly Assess Where You Are

One of the major principles I strongly embrace is to listen to your body and to adjust your program based on the feedback it is providing you. But it is also really good to have objective outside yardsticks. The following measures have been well established through many years of study; they have been time-tested and shown to be highly correlated to a reduced risk of disease.

The following seven factors are your signposts along the road to optimal wellness. Determine the status of these proven markers of health now, and you'll be able to track your progress and success in improving your health using the methods and principles in this book.

The seven clinically proven gauges I advise you to assess now and continue to monitor—every six months or so—are:

1. Fasting insulin level
2. Vitamin D level
3. Waist-to-hip ratio
4. Body fat percentage
5. Cholesterol and HDL ratios
6. Blood pressure
7. Uric acid level

While I don't normally recommend you run out to see your doctor, it is important to get your insulin, vitamin D, uric acid, and cholesterol levels tested, because it is simply impossible for you to know your levels without testing.[1] At the following sites, you can directly order your own tests: www.directlabs.com, www.saveonlabs.com, and www.healthonelabs.com.

When you see these measures start to change, you'll feel powerful, comfortable, confident, and psychologically ready to take continually better care of yourself. That's when life gets its sweetest: you can enjoy a sense of great physical and emotional well-being knowing you're heading toward your goals and knowing you can continue to change and improve your health.

Health Factor 1: Fasting Insulin Level

Insulin is a hormone produced in your pancreas that regulates the amount of sugar in your blood. Insulin is absolutely essential to staying alive. But the sad fact is that most of you reading this have too much and have developed insulin resistance. This state is pushing you toward chronic degenerative illness, and it's increasing the rate at which you age.

Most adults have about one gallon of blood in their bodies and are quite surprised to learn that in that gallon, there is only one teaspoon of sugar. If the total amount of sugar in your blood were to rise to one tablespoon, you would quickly go into a hyperglycemic coma and die.

Your body works very hard to prevent this by producing insulin to keep your blood sugar from rising dangerously high. Any meal or snack high in grain and sugar carbohydrates typically generates a rise in your blood glucose. To compensate, your pancreas secretes insulin into your bloodstream, which then lowers your blood sugar.

If you have been consuming a diet consistently high in sugar and grains, over time your body's insulin receptors have become "sensitized" to insulin and require more and more insulin to get the job done. Eventually, you become insulin resistant. If you don't change your diet, you'll likely also become diabetic and have a far higher risk of heart disease, stroke, cancer, and Alzheimer's.

Even worse, high insulin levels suppress two other important hormones—glucagon and growth hormone—that are responsible for burning fat and sugar and promoting muscle development, respectively. So insulin from excess carbohydrates promotes fat, then impairs your body's ability to burn that fat.

To find out your insulin levels, the test you need to ask for is a fasting blood insulin test. This test is done by just about every commercial laboratory, and is relatively inexpensive.

You can safely ignore the reference ranges from the lab, as they are based on "normals" of a population that has highly disturbed insulin levels. A normal fasting blood insulin level is below 5, but ideally you'll want to be below 3. Remember this must be a fasting test, as it has little value if you weren't fasting.

Health Factor 2: Vitamin D Level

Though it may seem inconvenient to go out and get a blood test to monitor your vitamin D, I can confidently say that it is one of the most important things you can do for your health (more on that in Healing Principle 5). Be sure to ask your doctor for the correct test, which is 25(OH)D, also called 25-hydroxyvitamin D. In most states you can also order the test without a doctor's order from the nonprofit website http://www.grassrootshealth.net/.

The optimal level of vitamin D you're looking for is around 50 to 70 ng/ml. When you get your results, if they're not in this optimal range, then make it your priority to get them there by following the principles in Healing Principle 5.

Health Factor 3: Waist-to-Hip Ratio

A large waist size is a powerful predictor of being unhealthy because it is a sign that too much intra-abdominal or visceral fat surrounds your liver, kidneys, intestines, and other organs. This layer of fat impairs your organs' ability to function properly and dramatically raises your risk of diabetes, stroke, and heart attack.

The classic presentation of too much visceral fat is the apple shape. This is the person with a chubby tummy, typically above the belly button. Contrast this with the classic pear-shaped individual, who has a slim waist and bigger buttocks and thighs and is far less likely to have large amounts of visceral fat. These general approximations are typically but not always true—you can be trim through the middle and still have too much visceral fat.

To accurately determine your waist-to-hip ratio use a measuring tape to measure around the smallest part of your torso—typically, just above the belly button. That is your waist size. Then measure around the largest part of your buttocks to get your hip measurement. Finally, divide your waist measurement by your hip size. That number is your waist-to-hip ratio.

Waist-to-Hip Ratio	Men	Women
Ideal	0.8	0.7
Low Risk	<0.95	<0.8
Moderate Risk	0.96–0.99	0.81–0.84
High Risk	>1.0	>0.85

If you don't like your number, know that this is one of the first factors that will change as a result of following the Healing Principles in this book.

Health Factor 4: Body Fat Percentage

Many experts believe that your body fat percentage is the most accurate measure of obesity. Just like it sounds, it is simply the percentage of fat your body contains, and it can be a powerful indicator of your health. No matter what body shape or size you are, excessive body fat has been strongly linked to chronic health problems like heart disease, diabetes, Alzheimer's, and cancer. Too little body fat is also problematic and can cause your body to enter a catabolic state, where muscle protein is used as fuel. A general guideline, from the American Council on Exercise, on healthy body fat percentages follows:

Classification	Women (% fat)	Men (% fat)
Essential Fat	10–13%	2–5%
Athletes	14–20%	6–13%
Fitness	21–24%	14–17%
Acceptable	25–31%	18–24%
Obese	32% and higher	25% and higher

Fat calipers are one of the most trusted and accurate ways to measure body fat. A skinfold caliper is a lightweight, handheld device that quickly and easily measures the thickness of a fold of your skin with its underlying layer of fat. Amazon has a good selection of them ranging from inexpensive ones for $5 to professional versions up to $200. Taken at very specific locations on your body, these readings can help you estimate your total percentage of body fat.

You can also use a digital scale that determines body fat, which is what I personally use, such as an EatSmart Precision GetFit Body Fat Scale. This is a bit quicker and easier to use as all you need to do is initially program it and step on it with bare feet then wait less than a minute to see your body fat percentage.

Although the absolute percentage that a body fat scale provides may be off, the direction you are moving your body fat (whether up or down) will be relatively accurate. This is an incredibly useful measure of whether you're nearing a healthy state or not. It's important to note that you don't need both a scale and a set of calipers—either one alone will tell you your body fat composition.

❧

A TRULY EFFORTLESS—AND FREE—WAY TO GAUGE BODY FAT PERCENTAGE

You can get a good approximation of your body fat percentage by comparing yourself to pictures you can easily find online by typing "body fat percentage pictures" on Google. You can get a rough guess where you are in just a few seconds with this approach.

Whichever method you choose, remember that it is *far* better to monitor your body fat percentage than your total weight, as the body fat percentage—not weight—is what dictates metabolic health or dysfunction.

Health Factor 5: Cholesterol and HDL Ratios

Most people are seriously confused about their cholesterol levels. This is because too much emphasis is placed on the importance of lowering your total cholesterol. This soft, waxy substance is found not only in your bloodstream but also in every cell in your body, where it helps to produce cell membranes, hormones, vitamin D, and bile acids that help you to digest fat. Cholesterol also helps in the formation of your memories and is vital for neurological function.

Your liver makes about 75 percent of your body's cholesterol. There are two primary types:

1. **High-density lipoprotein or HDL:** This is the "good" cholesterol that helps keep cholesterol away from your arteries and scavenges and removes LDL by transporting it back to your liver, where it can be processed. HDL also helps to repair the inner walls of your blood vessels that can become clogged with plaque. This all helps to prevent heart disease.

2. **Low-density lipoprotein or LDL:** This "bad" cholesterol circulates in your blood and, according to conventional thinking, may build up in your arteries, forming plaque that makes your arteries narrow and less flexible (a condition called atherosclerosis). If a clot forms in one of these narrowed arteries leading to your heart or brain, a heart attack or stroke may result. I now believe that LDL isn't "bad"; it's a necessary building block of your cell walls. In fact, there are two kinds of LDL cells—fluffy and large

and dense and small. Of these two types, only the smaller versions of LDL appear to be harmful. When LDL cells are compact, they are better able to penetrate damaged arterial walls and contribute to plaque and hardening of the arteries—two hallmarks of cardiovascular disease. Two things that contribute to the compaction of LDL cells are trans fats (from partially hydrogenated oils so prevalent in processed foods) and insulin.

Also making up your total cholesterol count are:

- **Triglycerides:** Elevated levels of this dangerous fat have been linked to heart disease and diabetes. Triglyceride levels are known to rise from eating too many grains and sugars, being physically inactive, smoking cigarettes, drinking alcohol excessively, and being overweight or obese.
- **Lipoprotein (a), or Lp(a):** Lp(a) is a substance that is made up of an LDL "bad cholesterol" part plus a protein (apoprotein a). Elevated Lp(a) levels are a very strong risk factor for heart disease. This has been well established, yet very few physicians check for it in their patients.

A far more important and practical predictor of cardiovascular risk than your total cholesterol level is actually the ratio of good cholesterol (HDL) to total cholesterol, along with the ratio of triglycerides to HDL. To determine your levels, you will need to work with your doctor to get a blood test. Please note that all these tests need to be done fasting, or the results will not be accurate or predictive.

Know that your total cholesterol number on its own will tell you virtually nothing about your risk of heart disease, unless it is 330 or higher. The following two percentages are far more potent indicators for heart disease risk:

- **HDL/Total Cholesterol Ratio:** It should be above 24 percent and ideally 30 or higher. It rarely gets above 50, but to the best of my knowledge, the higher the number the better. Levels below 10 percent are very dangerous and usually indicate an imminent cardiovascular event, like a stroke or a heart attack.

  It is important to note that some clinicians actually obtain this ratio by dividing the total cholesterol by the HDL (Total Cholesterol/HDL). In this case, the numbers should be lower. The cutoff point for a poor ratio would be any number greater than 4, with greater than 10 having serious problems. This number rarely drops below 2.

- **Triglyceride/HDL Ratio:** It should be below 2. The higher this number is, the worse your insulin control may be.

Health Factor 6: Blood Pressure

Hypertension is the medical term given to high blood pressure, and the condition is incredibly common—about 1 in 3 people have it. Hypertension is defined as blood pressure above 120/80. And it is diagnosed by taking your blood pressure with a blood pressure cuff. You can have this done at your doctor's office, or do it yourself with a home blood pressure kit.

Essentially one out of four blood pressure readings taken at a doctor's office are inaccurate due in part to what's known as "white coat hypertension"—when the stress of being at the doctor's office artificially elevates blood pressure.[2] Many people are given a prescription unnecessarily as a result.

The conventional medical approach to controlling high blood pressure is nearly always a drug. It's a dream come true for drug companies, but it only addresses the symptoms of the disease, not the cause, and keeps you a paying customer for life. You would be far better served by addressing the underlying cause, which is typically insulin resistance and obesity.

Although elevated insulin levels are one of the most common contributors to elevated blood pressure, it's also common for stress and anxiety to contribute to this problem.

Ideally your blood pressure should be at or under 120/80 without medication. If you are on medication, you will be delighted to know that eating a low-grain, high-quality-fat diet, as I will recommend in these pages, tends to normalize elevated blood pressures in the vast majority of people. After you begin my nutrition plan and follow it for several months, if you don't see an improvement in your blood pressure, seek out a natural health care professional to fine-tune your program.

Health Factor 7: Uric Acid Level

Uric acid is a normal waste product found in your blood. It has been known for some time that people with high blood pressure, excess weight, gout, or kidney disease often have high uric acid levels.

Uric acid functions both as an antioxidant and as a pro-oxidant once inside your cells. So, if you lower uric acid too much, you lose its antioxidant benefits. But if your uric acid levels are too high, it contributes to harmful damage, known as oxidation, to your cells, which then leads to inflammation. That's why you want to be sure your uric acid levels stay within a healthy range.

The ideal range for uric acid lies between 3 and 5.5 mg per dl. If your uric acid levels are higher than this, you are likely consuming too much sugar and grain carbohydrates, which are converted to sugar in your body (more on this in Healing Principle 3). In fact, the connection between fructose consumption and increased uric acid is so reliable that a uric acid level taken from your blood can actually be used as a marker for fructose toxicity.

I recommend that a uric acid level be a routine part of your blood screening.

Keep Track

Once you've determined the current state of your seven factors, jot them down in the chart on page 262. Recording your baseline there will make it easy for you to see your progress in one glance when you reassess these yardsticks in another three to six months.

Part Two

Help Your Body Fix Itself

Healing Principle 1

Drink Pure Water

At a Glance

✓ Making sure you drink enough pure water is one of the most important and powerful steps you can take for good health.

✓ Soda, diet soda, commercial fruit juices, and sports drinks will seriously disturb your body's metabolism.

✓ Tap water is better but is likely contaminated with toxins (like disinfection by-products) that are a thousand times more toxic than chlorine bleach.

✓ Filtered tap water can be an excellent, inexpensive, and easy source of fluid replacement.

✓ Because you are also exposed to these toxins when you bathe, investing in a water filter for your shower is a powerful way to reduce your toxic load.

✓ For Advanced Effortless Healing, the newest research points to structured water.

About two thirds of your body is made up of water—your cells, organs, muscles, and even your brain are approximately 70 percent water. The water in your body is the main delivery system for nutrients and oxygen, as well as the power behind its waste removal system. If there isn't enough water to flush away your toxic wastes, they will damage your body. Water also aids in energy production and keeps your joints lubricated. Water is absolutely imperative for your body to function. Go without food, and you'll last several weeks. Go without water, however, and you'll die within a few days. Clearly, water is something you need plenty of to function, especially since every day your body loses water through urine and sweat.

One of the most exciting aspects of this principle is that if you get the fluid/water replacement issue right, then you have taken one of the most important and powerful steps you can in owning your health. This is not an overstatement. You simply must have a high-quality source of water, or you will never achieve the health you seek. This applies not only to the water you drink but to the water you use while bathing.

Drink Up

Despite the consistent recommendations of health professionals to drink eight eight-ounce glasses of water per day, your daily water consumption should be based on your size and activity level. Chronic low-grade dehydration is common—most experts maintain that 70 percent of Americans aren't drinking enough water. There are many reasons: We're so busy and distracted by checking our smartphones, watching TV, or working at our computers that we no longer recognize, much less hear, our body's cues for more water. And we have a tendency to neglect the simplest things that contribute to health—like drinking water—and instead look for a miracle cure to treat fatigue or a fancy lip balm to treat chapped lips (both of which are signs that you are dehydrated). So many suffer from dehydration, often because they are simply unaware of its symptoms.

Are you one of them?

The major symptoms of dehydration are thirst, dry skin, dark-colored urine, and fatigue. But take a look at some commonly overlooked symptoms of chronic dehydration:

- Digestive disturbances, such as heartburn and constipation
- Frequent urinary tract infections and kidney stones
- Premature aging—more noticeable wrinkles, cracked or flaky skin
- High blood pressure
- Headaches

How Do You Know If You're Getting Enough Water?

Staying well hydrated is essential. But whether you actually need eight glasses of water or more every day is questionable, because an individual's hydration needs are so variable. So just *how much* water do you personally need to drink to replenish what you've lost?

Thirst Is Your Body's Cry for Water

Thankfully your body will typically *tell* you when it's time to replenish your water supply, because once your body has lost between 1 and 2 percent of its total water, your thirst mechanism usually lets you know that it's time to drink!

Since your body is capable of telling you its needs, using thirst as a guide to how much water you drink is one way to help ensure that your individual needs are met, day by day. It is possible to misread these signals and confuse feelings of thirst for hunger. Therefore it can be helpful to drink a glass of water when you notice yourself feeling thirsty or hungry. (If you drink a glass of water and are still hungry after ten minutes or so, then you'll know that cue is truly for food.) And if it's hot or exceptionally dry outside, or if you are engaged in exercise or other vigorous activity, you will require more water than normal. But again, if you drink as soon as you feel thirsty, you should be able to remain well hydrated—and avoid eating when you're not truly hungry—even in these cases.

A common myth is that if you're thirsty, you're already dehydrated. The reality is that it's not too late, and in fact, thirst is your body's way of telling you to drink water. If you feel a little parched, you're not at risk of becoming dangerously dehydrated. When you get thirsty, the deficit of water in your body is still fairly trivial—the thirst mechanism is a very sensitive gauge.

Keep in mind that there are two exceptions to this rule. As you get older your thirst mechanism tends to work less efficiently,[1] so older adults—over sixty-five—will want to be sure to drink several glasses of water daily, regardless of their feelings of thirst. And if you are someone who just doesn't recognize when you are thirsty, you will need to be mindful of drinking throughout your day. It can be difficult to gauge your body's hydration status simply through thirst—it's far more likely that you have gotten out of the habit of listening to your body's cues because you feel more urgency to sit at your desk and be productive than to walk to the water cooler and fill your glass. That's why it's important to monitor the signs your body is giving you about your level of hydration.

Urine Is Your Hydration Report Card

The color of your urine is a powerful visual aid and can help you determine whether you are getting enough water. As long as you are not taking riboflavin (vitamin B_2, found in most multivitamins), which fluoresces and turns your urine bright yellow, then your urine should be a very light-colored yellow. (If you are taking B_2, just stop for a day and observe the color of your urine.) If it is a deep, dark yellow, then you are likely not drinking enough water. If your urine is scant or if you haven't urinated in several hours, that too is an indication that you're not drinking enough.[2]

Soda: The Thirst Quencher?

You may not be aware of it, but **the average person in the United States drinks fifty-seven gallons of soda per year**. In my experience, the single most important health step the average person can take is to stop drinking any type of soda or sports drink and switch to pure water. If you're already there, then all you'll need to do is to improve the quality of the water you're drinking.

Though by now most people are aware that sodas are laced with processed sugars like high-fructose corn syrup and artificial sweeteners, many don't know that their favorite sports and vitamin drinks contain these sweeteners, plus a whole host of frightening extras: toxic chemicals like chlorine, fluoride, phthalates, BPA, and disinfection by-products (DBPs). DBPs are produced when the chlorine used to disinfect water reacts with organic materials in the water to form hundreds of different toxins that are a thousand times more toxic than the original chlorine.[3]

It is very easy to fall victim to savvy marketers and think you're drinking something healthy. It's even easier to get confused about the quality of your beverages if you aren't paying attention to the details, which is what happened to my friend Brenda.

Brenda is in her late fifties and very active, but she was about thirty pounds overweight. I did not know it at the time, but she was on a shopping bag full of prescription drugs for rheumatoid arthritis, depression, pain, and lack of energy. Her doctor never gave her any guidance on nutrition, but she thought she was eating a pretty healthy diet.

She was on her own in selecting what would be best for her to drink. Because she worked outdoors in the summer heat, she needed to drink a lot. One day she was drinking a sports drink because she thought it would give her more energy. However, the ingredients contained in this drink included nothing particularly drinkable: a patented flame retardant called brominated vegetable oil (BVO) as well as artificial sweeteners, artificial colorings, and loads of high-fructose corn syrup.

Unable to stop myself, the doctor in me took over. I quickly showed her the list of ingredients—which included glucose and fructose, glycerol esters of wood rosins, sucralose, and acesulfame K[4]—and explained to her that what she thought was a health drink was similar to soda, except it was worse, because it stimulates the body to crave even more sugary fixes. My guess is that Brenda is not alone, and that millions of people are similarly confused.

Fortunately, Brenda listened to me and started drinking filtered, structured water (more on that soon) from my home. After only a few months, with just this change, she lost almost thirty pounds, had more energy, and stopped taking nearly half the medications she was on.

Remember, the only step she took was to change the fluids she was drinking.

POISONS IN A BOTTLE

Before you reach for that soda, diet soda, sports drink, or enhanced water, familiarize yourself with some of the ingredients you're likely to imbibe. The most troublesome are artificial sweeteners. Consider aspartame, sold under the brand names NutraSweet and Equal. Diet cola, which often combines aspartame and caffeine, is a powerfully addictive beverage. These two agents create a unique combination of excitotoxins that can kill off some of your brain cells. However, before they do, they give you something akin to a buzz. It's the perfect plan to get you to go back to the store to buy another soda. And maybe a supersize soda—after all, it has *zero* calories, no matter how much you consume.

But not so fast. You are sipping your way into a trap.

Consider that aspartame causes formaldehyde to build up in your tissues,[5] which results in all sorts of potentially serious medical problems, including:

- Headaches
- Visual disturbances
- Migraines
- Autoimmune diseases like multiple sclerosis
- Seizures

- Cognitive problems
- Fatigue
- Symptoms similar to Parkinson's disease
- Symptoms similar to attention deficit disorder

The food industry claims that aspartame is safe. However, if you look at the studies that claim to support aspartame's safety, you will see that 90 percent of them were funded by the food and beverage industry. Independent aspartame studies tell a totally different story: 90 percent of them have found serious health problems related to aspartame.

Most people drink diet soda to keep weight off. However, a 2014 study published in the *American Journal of Clinical Nutrition* analyzed food and nutrition records that followed study participants for a period of ten years. It found that overweight and obese people drank significantly more artificially sweetened beverages than people of a healthy weight. It also showed that overweight and obese people who regularly drank these "diet" beverages consumed more calories from food

(continued on next page)

than overweight and obese people who drank beverages sweetened with sugar. The net effect: drinking diet soda leads to weight gain, not weight loss.[6]

Aspartame is just one toxic additive that has become an integral part of the beverages that line ever more aisles at grocery stores. (I wrote an entire book about the dangers of artificial sweeteners called *Sweet Deception*.) Here are some of the other ingredients to be avoided:

- **Propylene glycol.** This water-soluble, syrupy liquid is used as a base solution for various oils in packaged foods, fragrances, anti-freeze/coolants, and pharmaceutical products.[7] It also is a solvent for food colors and flavors. While the FDA has classified it as "generally recognized as safe" as an additive for food products,[8] exposure to it can potentially result in cell mutations and skin, liver, and kidney damage, if ingested in high enough amounts.[9] The Environmental Working Group (EWG) rates propylene glycol as a low-to-moderate hazard.[10]

- **Sucralose.** Previously listed as "safe" by the Center for Science in the Public Interest, this artificial sweetener, commonly known as Splenda, was downgraded to "caution" after a 2013 animal study linked it to a higher risk of developing leukemia.[11] It also has been implicated, either in clinical studies or on "Splenda sickness" blogs, as a cause of respiratory difficulties, migraines, gastrointestinal problems, heart palpitations, and weight gain. The list of reported problems is growing by the day.[12]

- **Acesulfame potassium (acesulfame K).** This artificial sweetener contains methylene chloride, which has been linked to kidney tumors, headaches, depression, nausea, mental confusion, liver effects, and visual disturbances, as well as cancer in humans.[13]

- **Food dyes.** These coloring agents have been connected to a variety of health problems, including allergic reactions, hyperactivity, decreased IQ in children, and numerous forms of cancer.[14]

• **Polysorbate 60.** This ethoxylated emulsifying agent is rated as a low-to-moderate health concern by the Environmental Working Group. It can be contaminated with ethylene oxide and 1,4 dioxane, two carcinogenic industrial pollutants.[15]

• **Brominated vegetable oil (BVO).** Another emulsifying agent, BVO is banned in more than one hundred countries, but in the United States it is added to about 15 percent of all sodas to prevent citrus flavoring from separating and floating to the surface.[16] This vegetable oil, typically derived from corn or soy, is bonded with the element bromine, and was first patented as a flame retardant. Bromines are common endocrine disruptors.[17]

> I am convinced that for the typical American, and maybe for you and many of your friends and family, the most important health step you can take is to stop drinking soda, sports drinks, or artificially flavored and sweetened waters and replace them with pure water.

How to Break the Soda Habit

If you are currently drinking soda and feel that its addictive pull will be hard to break, here are some tips on how to eliminate this beverage. Knowledge is power: learning that soda pumps your body full of sugars (or artificial sweeteners, which are equally if not more dangerous), but also promotes dehydration and typically reduces the amount of healing water you drink, may help you break away.

How do you do it?

One of the best ways to easily transition away from soda is to buy one of the home carbonating systems, such as Soda Stream, that will provide you with a pure, filtered, carbonated beverage you can bottle at home. Many people miss the bubbly sensation of soda, and drinking carbonated water can alleviate that longing. You can add lime or lemon or cucumber for flavor.

If you are drinking three or more cans of soda a day, you may develop a caffeine withdrawal headache, since most sodas are loaded with caffeine. The best way to know how quickly to reduce your intake is to listen to your body.

Reduce your intake to zero gradually, over a few weeks, lowering the amount you drink by a small amount every day until you stop. A good rule of thumb is to aim for a 5 to 10 percent reduction every day. So if you are drinking six 12-ounce cans (72 ounces) a day, you can reduce it by 3 to 7 ounces a day. At that rate you would be off soda in 10 to 20 days. Please remember that this is just a range. You may need to go more slowly if you are experiencing headaches.

If your cravings are simply too strong and you are unable to wean yourself off soda this way, you can try the extremely powerful energy psychology therapy called Turbo Tapping. It is an offshoot of EFT (Emotional Freedom Technique), which has helped many stop their addiction to this pernicious habit. Please refer to Healing Principle 8 for a basic introduction to this simple yet profound method.

Others to Eliminate

If you are searching for healthy water on the shelves of your grocery store, your head is likely swimming with all the options and competing claims each bottler makes. Here is your guide to the worst offenders.

Bottled Water

If you think you're getting a pure water from a bottle, don't be too sure: an independent test performed by the Environmental

Working Group found a whopping thirty-eight low-level contaminants in bottled water. Each of the ten tested brands contained an average of eight chemicals: DBPs, caffeine, Tylenol, nitrate, industrial chemicals, arsenic, and bacteria were all detected.[18]

Another concern is the bottle itself. Most plastic water bottles contain phthalates and BPA, which mimics hormones in your body.[19] I recommend drinking water from glass bottles whenever possible.

Functional Waters

The market has been flooded with "functional waters," fortified (supposedly) with everything from vitamins and minerals to electrolytes, oxygen, fiber, and even protein. Supermarket beverage aisles can entice you with a virtual sea of beverage choices—energy drinks, healthy teas, chia drinks, juices, vitamin waters, fitness waters, and sports/electrolyte concoctions in every imaginable color and flavor.

But if you take a look at the labels, you'll discover that the manufacturers are spiking your punch with a lot of unsavory ingredients, like high-fructose corn syrup and aspartame and many other substances capable of wreaking havoc on your body—*some of which are outright dangerous.* If you aren't already a label reader, *it's time you become one,* lest you fall prey to these clever marketing ploys. Flashy labels, pretty colors, and seductive scents are incredibly alluring, *especially to kids.*

Sports Drinks

As I covered in Brenda's story, sports drinks are a nutritional disaster. Very few people even benefit from this type of fluid replacement. A healthy alternative to sports drinks is to simply add a small amount of natural, unprocessed salt, such as Himalayan salt, to your regular drinking water. Typically a pinch or quarter teaspoon per liter is just fine. Unlike processed salt, natural salt contains many different minerals and trace minerals that your body needs for optimal function.

If you really do need fluid replacement from excessive sweating, then coconut water (which is loaded with natural minerals) and fresh fruit, not fruit juice, are far better choices. Be sure to limit your intake, however, to endurance exercises or environments where you are sweating more than a quart of water. Typically a quart of water weighs two pounds, so you can easily determine whether you need fluid replacement by weighing yourself before and after you exercise.

All Tapped Out

Likely you believe that tap water is a safe and healthy source of water. In the United States, at least, tap water is virtually pathogen free, and you will not get nasty infectious diarrhea from it, as you would in many countries around the world. While tap water is far superior to any type of soda, it is also generally loaded with a large number of toxic ingredients that may contribute to health problems.

Disinfection By-Products (DBPs)

Chlorine or chloramines are added to most municipal water supplies to sterilize the water. Chlorine itself is relatively safe, but it interacts with organic material in the water to form more than six hundred DBPs. These chlorinated organic chemical toxins include four primary compounds commonly referred to as trihalomethanes,[20] which, again, are minimally a thousand times more toxic than chlorine. In fact, trihalomethanes have *no* safe level,[21] which explains why DBPs, which have been linked to liver, kidney, and nervous system problems, are likely the worst toxins in most tap water in the United States.[22]

Fluoride

For many decades we've been told fluoride was essential for healthy teeth. We're now finding that this is not true. In fact, researchers from Harvard Medical School added fluoride to the list of top developmental neurotoxins in 2014.[23]

You may be surprised to learn that the fluoride that is added to our water supplies is actually hydrofluorosilicic acid—a hazardous waste product from the wet scrubbing systems of the fertilizer industry. Fluoride is the only drug that is forced as mass medication on the population with no control of dosing. In addition, 99 percent of all fluoride never touches your teeth. It literally goes down the drain (via your dishwasher, sinks, and tub), and into the environment.

Even with so little fluoride making it into our mouths, the CDC has admitted that due to the excess fluoride in our food and water 41 percent of adolescents now have dental fluorosis, a condition that occurs from an excess of fluoride.[24]

The United States is far behind the curve when it comes to fluoridation. In western Europe, 97 percent of the population drinks nonfluoridated water.[25] According to data gathered by the World Health Organization and the Fluoride Action Network, there is no discernible difference in tooth decay between developed countries that fluoridate their water and those that do not.[26]

Even in North America, water fluoridation has come under increasing scrutiny; since 2010, more than ninety U.S. and Canadian communities have voted to end water fluoridation.[27] The issue is heating up as more and more people begin to demand water that does not expose them to this highly toxic industrial waste product.

Many people assume that consuming fluoride is an issue that involves only your dental health. But nearly three dozen human studies and one hundred animal studies have shown that fluoride toxicity can lead to a wide variety of health problems, including:

- Increased lead absorption[28]
- Lowered IQ in children[29]
- Hyperactivity and/or lethargy[30]
- Muscle disorders[31]
- Gastroenterological problems[32]
- Arthritis[33]
- Dementia[34]
- Bone deformations and fractures[35]
- Thyroid disease and lowered thyroid function[36]
- Bone cancer (osteosarcoma)[37]
- Inactivation of 62 enzymes and inhibition of more than 100[38]
- Inhibited formation of antibodies[39]
- Genetic damage and cell death[40]
- Increased tumor and cancer rate[41]
- Disrupted immune system[42]
- Impaired glucose intolerance[43]
- Damaged sperm and increased infertility[44]
- Increased cardiovascular risk[45]
- Severe tooth enamel fluorosis, enamel loss and pitting, and delayed tooth eruption in children[46]

If you choose to use fluoride, then use it topically and heed to the warnings listed on poison control labels—as well as tubes of toothpaste—and do not swallow it![47]

**JOIN THE FIGHT TO GET FLUORIDE
OUT OF DRINKING WATER**

Water fluoridation is a form of mass medication that denies you the right to informed consent.

Fluoride is difficult to remove from drinking water once it's been added—very few water filters reduce it significantly. The only way to truly exercise your right to not ingest this medicine is to prevent it from being added to the water supply in the first place.

If you'd like to learn more and get involved in the effort to get fluoride out of the American water supply, join the Fluoride Action Network at fluoridealert.org.

Aluminum

You may have heard that aluminum increases your risk for Alzheimer's disease. But did you also know that the aluminum found in your municipal water supply can cause a wide variety of other health problems, including hyperactivity, learning disabilities, gastrointestinal disease, skin problems, Parkinson's, and liver disease?[48]

Arsenic

Arsenic, a poisonous element, is a powerful carcinogen. It has been linked to an increased risk of the development of several types of cancer.[49]

The Natural Resources Defense Council estimates as many as 56 million Americans living in twenty-five states drink water that contains unsafe arsenic levels. For more information, visit the website of the U.S. Geological Survey at http://water.usgs.gov/nawqa/trace/arsenic. It offers maps showing where and to what extent arsenic naturally occurs in groundwater across the United States. Arsenic is not easily removed by most carbon filters, but can be removed by reverse osmosis filters and distillation.

Prescription and OTC Drugs

Unwanted or expired prescription and over-the-counter (OTC) drugs that have been discarded in the trash or flushed down the toilet can end up in the public water supply. This practice has several possible outcomes:

- Drugs that were intended only for external application may be ingested. Or vice versa; you are exposed to the contaminants in water when you shower or take a bath.
- Some individuals are allergic to drugs found in the water supply.
- People are exposed to many combinations of drugs that have never been tested for safety when combined.
- Pregnant women are exposed to drugs that could potentially harm an unborn child.

Industrial Waste Products

In addition, chemical fertilizers and pesticides used by the farming industry are also washed into the water supply via rain runoff. Chemicals used in the controversial practice of fracking—which is used to harvest natural gas underground—can also find their way into your tap water.

Water Filtration Systems

To obtain water that is virtually toxin free, the best choice is to invest in a water filtration system. They come in several different types. Let's review them and weigh the pros and cons of each one.

Reverse Osmosis Filter

A reverse osmosis (R/O) filter will remove chlorine and the inorganic and organic contaminants in your water. It will also remove about 80 percent of the fluoride and most of the DBPs. But again, the best way to have fluoride-free water is not to put it in the first place, so join the Fluoride Action Network at fluoridealert.org, which is trying to remove it from our water supply.

Like distillation, R/O filtration creates fairly acidic water. And also like distillation, it strips the water of minerals.

The major drawback of R/O is the expense of installation. Typically a plumber is required. But a number of R/O systems don't require a plumber, which automatically cuts down on the cost.

The other major drawback is that the R/O filtration process is relatively slow: unless you have a pump to help force water through the membrane faster, it may take a few minutes to fill a glass of water. R/O systems can also be relatively inefficient. Many models will use five gallons of water to create one gallon of filtered water.

Cleaning may also become a problem. The systems usually use one- to five-gallon holding tanks, which have to be regularly cleaned so they don't become contaminated with mold. But a number of R/O systems have come on the market that have no holding tank. So you can store the water directly in a glass container, which can be regularly cleaned more easily.

Water Distillers

Distilled water is very pure and free of contaminants. But like R/O water, it has lost virtually all its beneficial minerals. Since water does not like this imbalance, it seeks to replace the lost minerals by using the ones in your body to fill the void, which can lead to mineral deficiencies. It is also acidic water and loses even more beneficial structure than R/O water. However, you can compensate by adding minerals back in with a pinch of natural Himalayan salt, which naturally contains minute levels of many minerals.

Carbon Filters

Granular carbon and carbon block filters are the most common types of countertop and under-counter water filters. The EPA recognizes granular activated carbon as the best available technology for the removal of organic chemicals like herbicides, pesticides, and industrial chemicals.

Granular carbon systems are far easier to use than R/O systems with holding tanks. But they don't filter the water as well, and most remove very little fluoride.

Whole-house systems are much larger than countertop models: they are about one-fourth the size of a typical water heater when installed—the larger the filter, the more toxins it removes.

They are typically installed close to the main water supply of the house. The inexpensive pre-filters are changed once a month or so based on the water quality in your area. The main primary filter will last for five years or more, depending on how much you use it. While this is a more expensive option, combined with a water-restructuring device, it will give you some of the healthiest water you can drink.

To get the highest-quality water in your home, use a whole-house carbon system and a R/O filter in the kitchen sink for drinking and cooking. It's not exactly cheap or effortless, I admit, but it's a boon for your health, as evidenced by Brenda's story.

Shower Filter When you take a shower, water comes in contact with your skin and also with your lungs, when you breathe in steam. When that water is contaminated, it can cause far more damage than if you drank it.[50] Shower filters are far less expensive than many drinking water filters. Another alternative is a whole-house water filter, which has the added benefit of removing contaminants from the water you use to brush your teeth, take a bath, and drink and cook with, too.

Installing a shower filter will significantly reduce your chemical exposure. For the rest of your life, it will spare your body in numerous ways. Your body won't have to detox those chemicals, your hormones won't be disrupted, and your risk of developing environmentally triggered diseases will be greatly reduced.

TIME TAKEN, TIME SAVED

Ideally, it would be best to install a whole-house water filter. However, if that's not feasible, installing a water filter for your shower will take about three hours—one hour to investigate the model, one hour to go to the store to purchase it (less if you buy it online), and one hour to install it (less if you hire someone to do it for you). And every few months, you will have to replace the filter, so let's add in another two hours for each year. Those three hours now (and two hours each year thereafter) will save you from inhaling and absorbing all manner of contaminants. By significantly reducing your chemical exposure—and when you calculate the compounds you won't be exposed to over the course of the rest of your life, it becomes a very significant amount—you'll be sparing your body in numerous ways. For starters, it won't have to work to detox those chemicals, your hormones won't be disrupted, and your risk of developing environmentally triggered diseases will be greatly reduced.

Water Filter Type	Cost
Countertop carbon filter	$36.99–$499.00
Whole-house carbon filter	$179.95–$2,039.00
Reverse osmosis filter	$76.47–$998.00
Distiller	$99.00–$3,141.60
Carbon shower filter	$14.08–$197.99

Healthy Drinks

Jazz Up the Taste of Your Water

If you don't like the taste of your water, here are a few ways to add flavor that will also impart health benefits:

- For a refreshing twist, add fresh lime or lemon wedges, slices of cucumber, or even peeled ginger root to your water.
- Try adding a drop or two of natural peppermint extract or a few crushed mint leaves from your herb garden.

- Use whole herbal tea extracts, and sweeten your drink with a safe, natural sweetener like stevia or lo han.
- Consider purchasing a machine to carbonate beverages at home.

Vegetable Juice

For the ultimate refreshing vitamin-rich drink, make up some green juice from fresh organic veggies. Don't add any fruits, except lemon or lime, due to their sugar content. (For more on juicing, see Healing Principle 2.)

Tea and Coffee

Tea is the better choice for many, but coffee can also be a healthy option. Tulsi (also known as holy basil) or hibiscus sweetened with some stevia are my personal favorites. Make sure both are organic. Use pure filtered water as your base. If you need a sweetener, use stevia or lo han instead of sugar—two natural choices I discuss further in Healing Principle 9.

| ADVANCED EFFORTLESS HEALING |

Structured Water

I left the best for last, because what I am about to discuss is one of the most exciting things that can effortlessly improve your health. I am referring to structured water or, as some call it, living water.

Structured water is physically different from what we typically drink as water: it has a different chemical structure. It is not H_2O, but H_3O_2. It is the type of water that occurs within our cells; it also occurs in many natural springs when a cold

mountain stream first comes bubbling out. This water has a negative charge and can hold energy, much like a battery, and it can
deliver energy too. Researchers believe it may provide the energy
for the electronegativity of your cells, which empowers them to
perform all their biological functions.

You can get an idea of why this works by looking at how an
infusion of rainwater can affect a lawn. If you have ever had a
lawn, you know that rainwater is superior to tap water sprinkled
on the lawn. This is largely related to the fact that rainwater is
structured and tap water is not.

In writing this book, I interviewed Dr. Gerald Pollack, who is
an international leader in the field of water research. He's a professor of bioengineering at the University of Washington and has
advanced our understanding of the physical structure of water
and its importance to human health. Dr. Pollack explained to
me that structured water molecules are more tightly organized
than those of typical water—think of a suitcase with clothes that
you've simply thrown in versus one where you've carefully rolled
and tucked the contents; the organized suitcase is more compact
and denser: you wouldn't have to sit on it to close the lid, as you
would with the disorganized one. Pollack hypothesizes that this
compactness makes structured water better suited to penetrate
our cell walls—it can get through smaller holes than a larger,
more typical water molecule can—and deliver hydration more effectively than regular water.[51]

Should You Drink Structured Water?

The best way to answer this question is to get some help from the
plant world. When we used structured water to grow our sprouts
in the Mercola.com offices, we consistently noticed a 30 to 40
percent increase in sprout harvest compared with plain filtered
water. You can have many theories on how or why something

should work, but ideally it is great to have a biological system to help us answer the question more conclusively.

According to the great science that is carefully detailed in Dr. Pollack's two books, structured water is the type of water many of our ancestors drank. There is clear biological support for its benefit with virtually no downside. So it is reasonable to conclude that it would be prudent to regularly consume structured water.

Ways to Add Structure to Your Water

If you are intrigued by the idea of drinking structured water, here are four ways to either find it or create it:

Raw, or juiced, vegetables. Fresh fruits and vegetables are loaded with structured water but tend to lose it once they are cooked or heated. So eat plenty of raw fruits and vegetables, or juice them.

Spring water. Water from deep sources, such as spring water, is another good source. The deeper the spring the better, as pressure is what structures the water. The mineral content of spring water also helps build structure.

Chilled water. Cooling water to about 39 degrees Fahrenheit appears to add some structure to it, although the molecules won't be as compact—and thus, as usable by your cells—as spring water or vortexed water. Even better: drink chilled spring water.

Vortexed water. The concept of vortexing water was based on observations from a nineteenth-century Austrian naturalist Viktor Schauberger. He found that the circular motion of vortexes adds structure and oxygen to water. Think of waves curling in on themselves and the flow of rivers and streams and the eddies contained with them. The swirling movement of water is also a key means of purification.

Other experts now believe that this motion gives the water molecules a tighter, more ordered structure. This may be one reason why swimming in flowing bodies of water, such as the ocean or mountain streams, is so revitalizing. You can now buy a vortexing machine that can transform your filtered water into structured H_3O_2. I have one in my home.

I believe the benefits of drinking structured water will become as popular as the benefits of getting plenty of vitamin D through regular sun exposure.

Your Effortless Action Plan

1. Stop drinking soda (including diet soda), sports drinks, and enhanced water and replace them with pure, clean water.

2. Invest in a high-quality water filtration system, for the most cost-effective source of clean water. If you can only afford one water filter, opt for a shower filter or a whole-house filter (which will also filter your shower water). If you can afford two, opt for a shower or whole-house filter and a R/O filter for your kitchen sink so that you can remove most fluoride from your drinking and cooking water.

3. If you need variety in your hydration, choose from organic tea and coffee, raw vegetable juices, and fresh coconut water.

4. To obtain even greater health benefits from water, seek out structured water. An effortless way: chill spring water, then drink up!

HEALERS	HURTERS
✓ Filtered tap water	✗ Soda
✓ Spring water	✗ Diet soda
✓ Filtered bathing water	✗ Sports drinks
✓ Chilled drinking water	✗ Fruit juice
✓ Organic tea and coffee	✗ Sweetened beverages (iced tea, lemonade, etc.)
✓ Carbonated water	
✓ Fresh, raw vegetable juice	
✓ Fresh coconut water	
✓ Vortexed water	

Healing Principle 2

Eat Your Veggies
(Four Effortless Ways to Eat More)

At a Glance

✓ The primary goal of an Effortless Healing eating plan is to normalize your insulin and leptin levels so that your body can once again effectively burn fat as a primary fuel.

✓ By adding significantly more vegetables and healthy fats to your diet, you will crowd out the processed foods, sugars, and grains that contribute to insulin and leptin resistance.

✓ Potassium and salt ratios are important to heart health.

✓ I recommend organic and/or locally grown vegetables: eating raw, juicing, fermenting, and sprouting.

The process of healing virtually every major disease, from cancer to diabetes to heart disease, has at its core the same basic approach: optimize your diet to improve your insulin and leptin sensitivity. This simple tactic will improve nearly every disease.

Even if you are basically healthy, eating to assist your body's receptivity to insulin and leptin will improve nagging conditions you might suffer from like constipation, fatigue, poor sleep, allergies, and a compromised immune system.

Your *best* strategy for improving your health is to choose the highest-quality foods. You want to eat a wide variety of whole, organic, and locally grown foods, primarily vegetables and high-quality fats. (See my version of the food pyramid below for more specifics.)

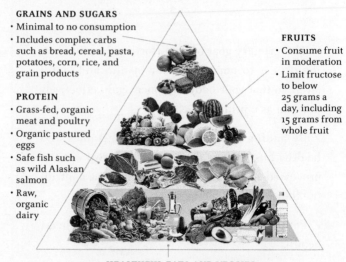

GRAINS AND SUGARS
- Minimal to no consumption
- Includes complex carbs such as bread, cereal, pasta, potatoes, corn, rice, and grain products

FRUITS
- Consume fruit in moderation
- Limit fructose to below 25 grams a day, including 15 grams from whole fruit

PROTEIN
- Grass-fed, organic meat and poultry
- Organic pastured eggs
- Safe fish such as wild Alaskan salmon
- Raw, organic dairy

HEALTHFUL FATS AND VEGGIES
- Healthy fats include coconuts, avocados, olive oil, butter, and raw nuts
- Raw, organic vegetables

You'll notice what's missing from this plan—most of the mainstays of the standard American diet, which consists of sugar, grains, and starchy carbs such as bread, pasta, potatoes, corn, and rice. I can hear the arguments already. How can arranging my diet in this way be effortless? At first blush, it may seem a huge undertaking to revamp your diet, particularly if you've been eating a grain-heavy feast of pasta, sandwiches, pizza, and French fries as the typical American has. But consider the success of one of my readers, Anna.

Anna was in her late thirties and experiencing an array of mysterious health issues, including an irregular heartbeat, digestive issues, strange rashes on her face, night sweats, painful periods, sinus headaches, and insomnia. Then she had triplets, and her symptoms only got worse. Anna's doctor suggested some supplements for her, but they didn't provide any noticeable relief.

When Anna took it upon herself to give up her reliance on grains and eat primarily vegetables and high-quality fats, all her ailments cleared up—even when she had three infants to care for. In addition, she lost weight (dropping several dress sizes), built muscle, radically increased her energy, and slept better than ever. When her husband asked if she missed pizza, Anna listed the benefits she's experienced to communicate that no, she didn't miss the bloating, belly fat, and laundry list of symptoms in the least.

Spending time nurturing yourself doesn't have to mean working hard and sweating bullets. I see it instead as a type of pampering. Choosing to take control of your health can take milliseconds; executing that choice may take longer, but time and effort aren't necessarily joined at the hip. When you're empowered to choose the foods that help your body run as it was designed to run, your body will reward you with a level of vitality that requires little to no effort to maintain, particularly compared to the time and energy you once had to spend on managing or suffering through problematic symptoms.

I'll talk more about why, how—and for how long—to wean yourself off grains in subsequent chapters. Here I want to focus more on the type of food you likely need to start eating much more of: vegetables.

Why Vegetables?

Vegetables are the food group that should take up the most room on your plate. To be more specific, fresh, minimally processed high-quality vegetables, ideally locally grown and organic. You should consume a majority of them raw.

It is very difficult to eat too many nonstarchy vegetables, as they have so much fiber, they will fill you up before you can overeat them. Because they are not calorie dense, they will typically comprise the largest portion of food on your plate. But if you are counting calories, which I don't personally do or advise, they may actually be only 10 to 25 percent of your total calories.

Nearly everyone would benefit from eating as many vegetables as possible to increase the amount of fiber, vital phytonutrients, and, most important, potassium, which counters the sodium in processed foods.

The Potassium-to-Sodium Ratio

Emerging evidence suggests that having a proper ratio of potassium to sodium in your food intake is crucial for improving your health. Although sodium is often blamed for hypertension, we are now beginning to see that hypertension is caused not simply by a high level of sodium but by a combination of too much sodium and—here is the underappreciated gem—too little potassium.[1]

Your body needs potassium not only to help regulate blood pressure but to maintain proper pH levels in your body fluids. Your body has evolved to require much more potassium than most of us take in today. According to a 1985 article in the *New England Journal of Medicine,* titled "Paleolithic Nutrition," our ancient ancestors got about 11,000 mg of potassium a day and about 700 mg of sodium.[2] This equates to a potassium-to-sodium ratio of nearly 16 to 1.

But in today's modern diet, daily potassium consumption averages about 2,500 mg and sodium intake hovers closer to 4,000 mg. A 16-to-1 ratio may be difficult to achieve, but consuming five times more potassium than sodium is very nearly effortless when you replace processed foods with vegetables. As a reward, you'll dramatically reduce your risk of dying from cardiovascular disease.

A 2011 federal study of sodium and potassium intake found that those at greatest risk for cardiovascular disease were those who got *too much sodium* combined with *too little potassium*. The study, published in *Archives of Internal Medicine,*[3] found that those who ate a lot of salt and very little potassium were more than twice as likely to die from a heart attack as those who ate about equal amounts of both nutrients.

Fresh vegetables are excellent sources of potassium. By eating more of them, you naturally reduce sodium intake by crowding out salty processed foods. If your diet doesn't provide you with adequate sources of potassium, consider taking a supplement.

Food Sources of Potassium	
Swiss chard	960 mg of potassium per 1 cup
Avocado	874 mg per cup
Spinach	838 mg per cup
Crimini mushrooms	635 mg in 5 ounces
Broccoli	505 mg per cup
Brussels sprouts	494 mg per cup
Celery	344 mg per cup
Romaine lettuce	324 mg per 2 cups

Are All Vegetables the Same?

Remember this important principle: vegetables are generally good, but not all vegetables are created equal. For example, increasing your vegetable intake with salads is a good start, but iceberg lettuce has minimal nutritional value. Red and green leaf lettuce, along with romaine lettuce and spinach, are far more nutritious options. Remember: the greener or darker the vegetable, the more nutritious it will typically be.

It's also important to eat primarily nonstarchy vegetables (think spinach and cucumber instead of potatoes), because the high-starch vegetables convert into glucose once you eat them, which then triggers your body's release of insulin. And remember, your primary goal in attaining optimal wellness is healing insulin and leptin resistance.

Additionally, finding organic vegetables is important. Your absolute best bet is to try to locate organic vegetables that have been grown locally, rather than those that have been shipped from across the country or overseas.

Conventionally farmed vegetables are not your best choice. Organic vegetables are a much better option. But if you can't obtain organics, any vegetable is better than no vegetable! Getting all your vegetables from conventionally farmed sources would be better for your health than eating no fresh vegetables at all. Just take extra care with nonorganic vegetables: wash them thoroughly, and remove peels and cores when possible, to minimize your exposure to pesticides.

Maybe you don't know the full picture of why it's really worth it to invest in organic for your health. USDA Organic farmers (and many small, local organic farms working without certification) must use different standards when growing vegetables. These standards include restricted use of:

- Pesticides
- Synthetic fertilizers
- Sewage sludge
- Genetically modified organisms (GMOs)
- Ionizing radiation

The EPA considers 60 percent of herbicides, 90 percent of fungicides, and 30 percent of insecticides to be carcinogenic, and most of them are damaging to your nervous system as well.

Buying your vegetables from a local organic source—or better yet, growing them yourself—is the ideal way to ensure that they are both fresh and high-quality.

If you are unable to obtain organic vegetables, you can rinse nonorganic vegetables in a sink full of water with 4 to 8 ounces of distilled vinegar for 30 minutes. This will help remove some of the pesticides but certainly not all, as some like glyphosate (Roundup) are actually integrated inside the cells of the plant.

When storing fresh produce, be sure to squeeze as much air as you can out of the bag that holds the vegetables, then seal it. The bag should look as if it is vacuum-packed. The reason is that fruits and vegetables release ethylene gas after they are harvested. Ethylene gas accelerates ripening, aging, and rotting.

Removing as much air as possible from the bag can decelerate this process. I hold the bag against my chest and run my arm over the bottom of the bag to the top, which bleeds the air out of the bag. You can also use vacuum sealer systems like the Food-Saver, which has an attachment to create vacuums in simple Ball jars.

By following this simple tip, you will double or triple the normal storage life of your vegetables.

The Best Vegetables for Good Health

HIGHLY RECOMMENDED VEGETABLES	
Asparagus	Escarole
Avocado (actually a fruit)	Fennel
Beet greens	Green and red cabbage
Bok choy	Kale
Broccoli	Kohlrabi
Brussels sprouts	Lettuce: romaine, red leaf, green leaf
Cauliflower	Mustard greens
Celery	Onions
Chicory	Parsley
Chinese cabbage	Peppers: red, green, yellow, and hot
Chives	Tomatoes (also technically fruits)
Collard greens	Turnips
Cucumbers	Spinach
Dandelion greens	Sprouts
Endive	Zucchini

USE SPARINGLY DUE TO HIGH CARBOHYDRATE LEVELS	
Beets	Jicama
Carrots	Winter squashes
Eggplant	

VEGETABLES TO AVOID	
Corn (really a grain but many consider it a vegetable)	Potatoes

Secrets to Effortless Vegetable Consumption

There are four main ways to make eating this many vegetables easy, delicious, rewarding, and fun. They are:

- Eating raw
- Juicing
- Fermenting
- Sprouting

Eating Raw

If you are intimidated by the thought of cooking piles of vegetables, take heart—by eating your veggies raw, you only need to wash and slice them; you won't have to also dirty a pan or take the time to cook them.

Why is eating raw food so important? Food contains many important micronutrients. Cooking and processing it can destroy these micronutrients by altering their shape and chemical composition. In fact, malnutrition—nutrient deficiencies—from consuming a highly processed diet is one reason many people cannot lose weight, because it leads to overeating. If you're consistently feeling hungry, you're likely not getting sufficient amounts of the nutrients your body needs to thrive.

Cooking foods at high heat can also produce unhealthy byproducts, such as acrylamide (a cancer-causing and potentially neurotoxic chemical)[4] and thermolyzed casein (a potentially carcinogenic dairy protein that has been linked to colon cancer).[5]

On a more holistic note, for optimal health you also need the live "sun energy" that's available only in raw, uncooked foods. The more light a food is able to store, the more nutritious it is.

While you can—and should—absorb the sun's healing energy through your skin (see Healing Principle 5), you can also take it in via your food, especially organically grown fresh vegetables, which store it in the form of biophotons.[6]

Bio-What?

Biophotons are a very-low-frequency emission of light, also known as "ultraweak photon emissions." Every living organism—including plants, animals, and humans—emits biophotons from its cells. It is thought that the higher the level of light energy a cell emits, the greater its vitality.

Cooking food is believed to dramatically weaken the biophotons in a food, and to lessen the potential for the transfer of that energy to the individual who consumes it.

You have likely heard of the raw food style of eating, wherein no food in the diet is heated above 118 degrees, so that the nutrients in the food aren't damaged. While some circumstances may merit this big of a shift in how you eat, the average person has a simpler way to consume more biophotons: to eat more raw veggies.

The trick to doing it effortlessly is to stock your vegetable drawer with the best-quality produce you can find. Cutting the vegetables up into snackable portions will make it easy for you to reach for them in moments of hunger, or bring them with you for a healthy snack on the go.

Juicing: Killing Two Birds with One Stone

Regularly consuming fresh vegetable juice will help you get more nutrients from vegetables. And it will easily help you reach the goal of eating at least 30 percent (and up to 50 percent or more) of your diet raw. As an added bonus, fresh vegetable juice is also an excellent source of structured water, which is covered in Healing Principle 1.

Juicing is a simple and easy way to virtually guarantee you will reach your daily target for vegetables. Beyond that, I am firmly convinced that the benefits of juicing are key to a radiant, energetic life and truly optimal health.

I first became excited about juicing when I treated a patient who was in her seventies but looked like she was in her forties. She attributed most of her youthful appearance to juicing. I decided to try it and have been juicing regularly ever since. I typically consume from a pint to a quart of green juice most days.

TIME TAKEN, TIME SAVED

Washing, slicing, and storing several different types of raw veggies will take at most twenty minutes after you get home from the grocery store. By doing them all at once, you'll avoid having to spend several minutes doing it every time, in the following days, that you need a snack or side dish. And skipping the cooking will save you even more time—at least ten minutes of cooking and a few minutes of washing pots. Beyond that, eating vegetables raw instead of cooked will supercharge the nutrition you receive from them, and it will contribute to your lifelong health.

Benefits of Juicing

You will want to incorporate vegetable juicing into your optimal health program for three main reasons:

- **Nutrition.** Juicing will help you absorb far more of the nutrients from the vegetables. As a result of making less-than-optimal food choices over many years, many of us have impaired digestion: our body's ability to absorb all the nutrients from the vegetables is limited. Juicing helps to "pre-digest" them, so you will receive most of their nutrition, rather than having it go down the toilet.
- **Convenience.** While juicing does require some prep work—you do need to clean and chop the vegetables—you can juice an entire day's worth of vegetables in one stint. You can then store any servings you don't consume right away in glass jars in the fridge. (Fill the jars to the very top to minimize the amount of air in the jar, which can oxidize and damage the juice.) They'll be perfect for grabbing and going. Just make sure to drink the juice within twenty-four hours—the fresher the juice, the more nutrients and benefits it will provide you.
- **Variety.** With juicing, you can add a wider variety of vegetables to your diet. Many people eat the same salads every day, which promotes boredom and increases your chance of developing an allergy to a certain food. But with juicing, you can drink a wide variety of vegetables that you might not normally enjoy eating whole.

Considerations

As you start on your juicing journey, keep a couple of considerations in mind:

Avoid Using Juice as a Complete Meal Unless you are undergoing some special fasting or detoxification program, it is probably unwise to use juicing as a meal replacement. Vegetable juice has very little protein and virtually no fat, so by itself, it is not really a complete meal. It should be used in addition to your regular meal, not in place of it. While juice offers a concentrated source of nutrients, it doesn't provide the beneficial fiber present in vegetables, which is important for nourishing your gut bacteria (more on this in Healing Principle 6). Ideally, you should consume it with your meal or as a between-meal snack.

Listen to Your Body Start by juicing vegetables that you enjoy eating non-juiced. The juice should taste pleasant—not make you feel nauseous. Listen to your body when juicing. Your stomach should feel good all morning long. If it is churning or growling or generally making its presence known, you probably juiced something you should not be eating. Some herbs and dark leafy greens are more likely to cause this. All you need to do to confirm that a suspected vegetable is a problem for you is to eliminate it and see if the symptoms disappear. If removing the vegetable solves the problem, then reintroduce it and see if the symptoms recur. If so, then you know that this is one food you should avoid or consume only in small quantities and only occasionally.

Limit Fruits You can certainly juice fruits too, but if you are overweight, have high blood pressure, diabetes, or high cholesterol, limit using fruits until you normalize these conditions. It would be *far* better to use lemons or limes than carrots, beets, or apples, which have significantly more fructose than lemons or limes. (For more on the perils of consuming fructose, see Healing Principles 3 and 9.)

Totally Juiced—Getting Started

Here are a few simple ideas to get you set up and help you enjoy the benefits of juicing quickly. (For a more complete guide to juicing, visit http://mercola.fileburst.com/PDF/JuicingGuide.pdf.)

Choose the Right Equipment Many people initially think juicing will be a real chore, but the majority are pleasantly surprised that it is actually fast and easy. Having the right tool for the job is important. If you are new to juicing, I recommend a midpriced juicer. Cheap centrifugal juicers break easily, produce low-quality juice, and are very loud, which may contribute to hearing loss. They also don't last very long. My favorites are the twin-gear juicers, like the juicer available for sale on our site. They are relatively fast and easier to clean.

Choose Pesticide-free Veggies Choose organic whenever possible. Some conventionally grown vegetables are worse than others and should be avoided, including these from the Environmental Working Group's 2013 list of most contaminated produce:

- Celery
- Cucumber
- Hot peppers
- Spinach
- Kale
- Collard greens
- Sweet red peppers

Start Your Juicer! Please note that the steps listed below are intended for those who are new to juicing, so that they have a pleasant experience with it. But even a beginner can start experimenting with some of the more bitter greens early on, using ¼ to ½ of a lime or lemon to effectively counter their bitterness.

Most fruits are best eaten whole, and in moderation, as they are not the same fruits our ancient ancestors ate. Rather, they have been bred over time to contain more fructose as we've continued to cater to our sweet tooth.

STEP 1: If you are new to juicing, I recommend starting with these vegetables, as they are among the easiest to digest and tolerate.
- Celery
- Fennel (anise)
- Cucumbers

These three aren't as nutrient dense as the dark green leafy vegetables. In the few days or weeks that it takes you to adjust to these three vegetables, you can start adding the more nutritionally valuable but less palatable vegetables into your juice.

STEP 2: When you've acclimatized yourself to juicing, you can start adding these vegetables:
- Red leaf lettuce
- Green leaf lettuce
- Romaine lettuce
- Endive
- Escarole
- Spinach

STEP 3: When you're ready, move on to adding herbs to your juicing. Herbs also make wonderful combinations, and these two work exceptionally well:
- Parsley
- Cilantro

Be cautious with cilantro, as many people cannot tolerate it as well. So start off with a few sprigs and work your way up from there. Use a few tablespoons if you have no side effects and enjoy the taste. If you are new to juicing, hold off on the cilantro. Herbs are more challenging to consume, but they are highly beneficial.

STEP 4: These greens are bitter, so start with a few smaller leaves at a time:
- Kale
- Collard greens
- Dandelion greens
- Mustard greens

When purchasing collards, find a store that sells the leaves still attached to the main stalk. If they are cut off, the vegetable rapidly loses many of its valuable nutrients.

Make Sure Your Juice Tastes Great To make your juice taste terrific, try adding:

LIME OR LEMON: Add a half to a whole lime and/or lemon for every quart of juice. You can actually juice the skin, if you want to avoid the hassle of peeling them.

CRANBERRIES: Add some fresh cranberries if you enjoy them. Cranberries have five times the antioxidant content of broccoli, which means they may protect against cancer, stroke, and heart disease. In addition, they are chock full of phytonutrients and can help women avoid urinary tract infections. Limit cranberries to about 4 ounces or half a cup per pint of juice.

FRESH GINGER: Ginger is an excellent addition if you enjoy the taste—it will give your juice a little kick! As an added bonus, researchers have found that ginger can have dramatic effects on cardiovascular health, preventing atherosclerosis, and helping prevent the oxidation of low-density lipoprotein (LDL).[7]

Clean Your Juicer Properly We all know that if a juicer takes longer than a few minutes to clean, we'll find excuses not to juice at all. I find that using a toothbrush works well on the metal grater. If you buy a high-quality juicer, the whole process should only take about five minutes, tops. Whatever you do, you need to clean your juicer immediately after you juice to prevent any remnants from contaminating your juicer; the most significant concern is mold growth.

For a more complete guide to juicing, visit juicing.mercola.com.

Fermenting: Another Great Way to Eat More Vegetables

Fermented vegetables offer two benefits in one package—they are a great way to consume more vegetables, and they deliver a healthy amount of beneficial bacteria that promote digestion and immunity.

A Beneficial-Bacteria Primer

Experts now believe that the ecosystem in your gut, on your skin, and throughout your body is one of the most complex on the planet. The type and quality of the foods you eat, by increasing the beneficial bacteria in your gut ecosystem, have an enormous influence on your health. Eating fermented foods is one of the simplest and least expensive strategies to increase gut bacteria.

Cultured foods such as yogurt, some cheeses, and sauerkraut are good sources of natural, healthy bacteria, provided they are not pasteurized.

I am a major proponent of fermenting vegetables at home—it's fairly easy, it's fun, and it's extremely cost effective. Fermented vegetables can provide your body with the same number of good bacteria as an entire bottle of high-potency probiotics, at a fraction of the cost. You can purchase probiotic supplements for $20 a bottle—or even $100 for some brands—but you can get the same benefits from fermented vegetables for a small fraction of that amount.

To learn more about the powerful benefits of fermented foods, and to discover the recipe we use to make fermented vegetables at our home office outside Chicago—where we offer fresh vegetable juice, these veggies, and organic lunches to all our employees—turn to Healing Principle 6.

A Caveat

If you are not used to eating fermented vegetables, it is best to start slowly so you don't kill off large numbers of bad bacteria all at once. They release toxic by-products when they die, which can trigger headaches, bloating, and general discomfort. Typically a half-teaspoon is a wise starting point. Work your way up gradually to a few tablespoons per day. Fermented vegetables are best consumed as a condiment rather than eaten by themselves. Be careful in purchasing fermented foods at your local supermarket, as many are pasteurized—a process that negates many of the intended benefits.

| ADVANCED EFFORTLESS HEALING |

Sprouting: Grow Your Own Sprouts

S prouts are some of the most nutrient-packed foods you can eat. They can have from ten to thirty times the nutritional content of even the organic vegetables grown in your own garden.

Nearly anyone can grow sprouts, even a student in a college dorm room, as it requires hardly any space. It really is quite simple and does not take more than a few minutes of your time, daily. You can grow them from seed to harvest in ten days—even in the middle of winter.

And it's inexpensive—growing a pound of sprouts at home usually costs less than a dollar. You can purchase sprouts from many health food stores, but they typically cost $20 to $30 a pound, and they won't be as fresh or tasty as when you grow them yourself.

Sunflower and pea sprouts top the list of nutrient-dense sprouts—and their taste is more palatable to many people than alfalfa and broccoli. Other seeds you can use would be mung bean, clover, radish, watercress, brassica, and wheatgrass (which is primarily for juicing, not for eating). They are all simple and rewarding to grow on your own.

Growing your own sprouts is an empowering activity that helps you and your family to take control of your health. Kids particularly enjoy the process, as they can see the entire transition, from seeds to four-to-eight-inch sprout, take place in as little as one week.

How to Grow Your Own Sprouts

The following instructions can be adapted to grow any sprouts. My recommendation is to start with sunflower sprouts, as they give you the most volume, taste delicious, and are loaded with dense nutrition for the ridiculously small effort you invest. You can certainly sprout other seeds for variety, but most people come back to sprouting sunflower seeds.

Procure Your Seeds The first step is to obtain some high-quality sunflower seeds (ideally organic, black, and unhulled) for sprouting—the package should say something to the effect of "sprouting seeds." It is best to get organic seeds so they are free of chemicals. A good starting amount is about one 8-ounce cup of seeds. We sell sprouting kits at Mercola.com to make this easier, but you can get the materials from many places online or even locally.

Procure a Planting Container or Tray You will need a container that is flat and about two inches deep. Or use a potting tray with drainage holes that is 10 inches square—enough space to grow one to one and a half pounds of sprouts. If you're growing sprouts for a number of people, you'll likely want to use a 10-by-20-inch tray. The smaller trays do allow you to harvest the freshest sprouts possible, though. These trays can be obtained online or from your local garden shop, and they're relatively inexpensive. If you're using a potting tray, you'll also need a larger drainage tray without holes, so that the water you use to water your seeds will drain into the other tray and not all over your kitchen counter.

Soak and Rinse Soak your seeds in filtered water for 6 to 8 hours. The easiest is to place the seeds in water just before going to bed and drain them in a mesh strainer when you wake up in the morning. Plastic Easy Sprouters are available, which make the soaking and rinsing much easier.

After soaking, rinse the seeds a few times over the course of twenty-four hours or so. At this point, you should see a tiny little white sprout coming out of many of the seeds.

Plant the Seeds You will need a container that is flat and about two inches deep. I use a potting tray with drainage holes that is 10 inches by 10 inches—enough space to grow one to one and a half pounds of sprouts.

The tray with the soil in it should have drainage holes and that should be put into a larger tray with no holes to catch any water that flows out.

Fill your container with about an inch of high-quality potting soil. I prefer to use a biochar compost blend. It is necessary to fill the tray only halfway up as the sprouts do not require a full tray of soil. If using a potting tray, place it inside of a larger drainage tray without holes, so that the water you use to water your seeds will drain into the bottom tray and not all over your kitchen counter. Make sure the soil is level. An easy way to do this is to level the soil with your hands, and then use another tray to firmly press the soil down.

Plant the Sprouted Seeds Stagger the planting of the seeds, depending on how much you and your family consume, to optimize the timing of your sprouts so you are always harvesting fresh sprouts. If you are growing them just for your own consumption, planting new seeds every four to five days may be sufficient. If your family is going through a tray a day, you will need to plant a new tray every day.

To stagger your planting, spread one-third to one-half of a cup of soaked and rinsed seeds over one-third or one-half a 10-by-20-inch tray, spreading the seeds evenly over the potting soil. After you have spread the seeds, add enough water to fully moisten all the seeds, but not so much that the seeds are sitting in standing water.

Make certain that you don't pour so much water into the tray that it pools, as that can contribute to mold growth, especially in the summer months. You will have to play with the exact amount, but it should be easy to figure it out after a few tries. It typically is about 2 cups of water for a 10-by-10-inch tray on the first day of watering, and 1 cup a day after that.

After a few days plant the remainder of the tray so you have a constant supply ready. Monitor the seeds every day during the ten-day growing period. It only takes a minute or so to water them, but if you leave home for a few days and fail to water them, they will die.

Challenge Them The next step is not obvious, but it is really important. Sprouts that are planted in the ground have to exert energy to go through the soil. If you don't provide this challenge for them (which potting soil doesn't), they will not grow as well.

Put a board or, even better, a piece of tile that covers the entire tray and lies directly on top of the seeds. And here is the key: put some weight on top of the board or tile so that it covers the whole tray. Five to 10 pounds will work just fine. Keep the weight on for two to three days, until the sprouts start pushing the board or tile up. A 10-by-10-inch paving stone works well; the strength of the little sunflower sprouts will surprise you!

Water Just Enough Give the sprouts about a cup of water a day until you harvest them. If you are in a hot and humid environment, it is possible you might get some mold. One way to limit this is to use a bit less water and make sure air can circulate around the sprouts. A gentle breeze is all that is needed. You really don't need to expose the sprouts to sunshine until about twenty-four hours before you harvest them.

If you are growing them indoors in the winter, sunshine through your window will work just fine. However, if you don't give them enough water, or if they are in the sun, they will tend to wilt and drop over. Don't worry—they aren't dead. All they need is some water; take them out of the sun or heat, and in twelve hours they will perk right back up.

Harvest Use a sharp pair of scissors, and cut the sprouts close to the soil level. Harvest only what you are going to eat so they are maximally fresh, but they should all be harvested within fourteen days of soaking the seeds.

Ideally, eat your sprouts immediately after harvesting, but you can store them in the fridge for five to seven days. Again, it's best to use a smaller tray so you can harvest them more frequently.

After you finish harvesting the sprouts, add the soil, cut stems, and roots to your compost pile, if you have one. That way, you can reuse it in a few weeks to grow another batch of sprouts. If you put the soil with the cut sprouts and roots into a compost pile or bin, be sure to break it up first so it will decompose more rapidly.

If you don't want to compost the soil, simply discard it on some plants outdoors that you want to help, as they will all welcome the healthy compost treat.

You can reuse your potting trays. Just be sure to wash them after each use with soap and water.

Your Effortless Action Plan

1. *Make local, whole, and organic vegetables the largest component of your diet (by volume—not by calories).*

2. *Seek to eat at least 50 percent of your vegetables raw.*

3. *Drink green juice (from fresh organic vegetables) several times a week.*

4. *Prioritize eating fermented vegetables for their health-promoting probiotic content.*

5. *Supercharge your nutrient intake by regularly eating sprouts. Try growing your own for truly effortless (and inexpensive) superfood nutrition.*

HEALERS	HURTERS
✓ High-water-content vegetables	✗ Starchy vegetables (particularly if you are insulin and/or leptin resistant)
✓ Raw vegetables	✗ Cooked vegetables
✓ Fermented vegetables	✗ Processed foods—chips, cookies, muffins, crackers, most packaged snacks
✓ Fresh vegetables	
✓ Vegetable juice	✗ Fruit juice
✓ Sauerkraut and kimchee	
✓ Sprouts	

TIME TAKEN, TIME SAVED

It may seem like a chore or even a punishment to eat more vegetables. But since you only have to wash and chop them (and even the chopping is optional), vegetables truly are nature's convenience foods. And while you're saving time on cooking and cleaning pots, you'll also be helping your body find its way back to balance, where insulin and leptin resistance disappear and Effortless Healing begins.

Healing Principle 3

Burn Fat for Fuel

At a Glance

✔ When it comes to losing weight, *when* you eat is just as important as *what* you eat.

✔ Breakfast really may not be the most important meal of the day, and it could be *adding* to your weight problem.

✔ Eating only during an eight-to-ten-hour window each day will help you burn fat and dramatically improve many markers of good health.

✔ For Advanced Effortless Healing, skip breakfast and work out while in a fasted state.

Two-thirds of Americans are overweight, and typically at any given time, more than 75 million are on diets seeking to lose weight. Sadly, over time, most of those diets fail and many people actually gain more weight than they lose.

The problems with carrying excess weight are more than simply aesthetic. At the root of obesity is a metabolic dysfunction—namely, insulin and leptin resistance (more on these in a moment). This develops as a result of consuming too many sugars and grains, then triggers the body to hold on to more weight.

These metabolic disorders go hand in hand with many of the chronic diseases that are plaguing Americans in record numbers—including diabetes, heart disease, high blood pressure, dementia, and cancer.[1] It has gotten to the point that one in five American deaths is associated with obesity, according to a 2013 Columbia University study.[2]

In this and the next Healing Principle, I'll share with you my two most effective strategies for correcting the metabolic imbalances that are at the root of obesity and so many chronic diseases. They will help you lose weight in a way that does not feel like deprivation or even sacrifice and that you can maintain over the course of your lifetime. Even if you aren't looking to lose pounds and/or belly fat, these strategies will also help you stay healthy and avoid chronic disease.

But to really rewire your thoughts on what it means to be on a "diet" and to "eat healthy," I first want to bust some of the most pervasive and harmful nutritional myths.

Major Myth 1: A Calorie Is a Calorie Is a Calorie

The first "rule" of dieting I'd like to dispel is the one that says your weight is the result merely of simple math: the calories you eat, minus the calories you burn. After all, a calorie is just a calorie.

Wrong.

Your lifestyle choices over the long term are the key to dietary success. Moreover, a reduced-calorie diet is difficult for most people to maintain, so even if your weight comes off, it generally returns when you resume your typical eating patterns.

If the calories you consume primarily come from sugar and grains—bread, pasta, rice, cookies, even fruit—you're conditioning your body to burn sugar as its primary fuel. When you consume sugar or grains, your body stores the sugar as glycogen in your liver and muscles. After the glycogen store is filled, any additional sugar you eat is converted to fat for long-term energy usage.

Foods high in sugar and grains will satiate your current hunger, but they can also set you up for metabolic disasters like obesity, fatigue, diabetes, and heart disease, and they can fuel excess body fat and obesity-related diseases.

Remember, when you eat sugar, your body releases insulin and leptin. These hormones play a key role in regulating your energy intake and expenditure, cuing it either to store the energy or to release your energy reserves. Eventually, if your body develops a resistance to insulin and leptin, you will require more and more of them to do their job. Your body will no longer hear its own signals to stop eating, burn fat, or pass up sugary foods. If you are insulin resistant, then eating even small amounts of fruits or grains can be a problem for you.

The result?

You stay hungry. You crave sweets. And your body stores even more fat, particularly around your belly. Other common ailments that develop as a result of insulin and leptin resistance are:

- Excess weight
- High blood pressure

- Diabetes
- Abnormal cholesterol ratios
- Cancer

Wouldn't it be nice to have an effective strategy that works without having to wrestle with your body's sugar craving and count calories all day long?

Thankfully, that is precisely what effortless eating offers.

Major Myth 2: High-Fat Diets Are Bad for You

Your body can burn either sugar or fat for fuel. Most of us have weeks' worth (and some many months') of fat stored to burn as fuel, but nearly all of us have only about twelve hours of sugar to burn.

After that twelve-hour window, your glycogen stores become depleted. When you regularly eat three meals a day, your body's glycogen stores are never fully emptied, and your body learns to rely on sugar as its primary fuel. You likely feel a frequent and urgent hunger to replace your sugar stores, because your body requires regular fuel, and if you can't access your fat stores, then you need to rely on using sugar as a fuel. Your body has essentially forgotten how to burn fat because it simply has no need to do so when you are in constant feast mode and have full glycogen stores.

One of the ways you can teach your body to start burning fat is to eat substantially more healthy fats, like coconut oil, olive oil, olives, butter, eggs, avocados, and nuts (more on this later in this chapter).

In fact, even though this may sound heretical, if you are insulin or leptin resistant, you could healthfully get as much as 50 to 75 percent of your daily calories from healthy fats. While this may sound like a lot, consider that, in terms of *volume,* the largest portion of your plate would be *vegetables,* since they contain so few calories. Fat, on the other hand, tends to be very high in calories. This idea is based on exciting research done by Dr. Thomas Seyfried and his work in the treatment of intractable seizures and cancer.[3]

The first step to teaching your body to make the switch from burning sugar to burning fat is to change the types of food you eat. Once you start to get the majority of your daily calories from vegetables and healthy fat, you will gently remind your body how to burn fat as fuel, and over a short time you will regain this important ability. But—and here is the shocker—*when* you eat is just as important, maybe even more, than *what* you eat.

WORKOUT
(7AM–11AM)

FAST (7AM–11AM)	EAT (11AM–7PM)	FAST (7PM–11PM)	SLEEP (11PM–7AM)

| 8 AM | 10 AM | 12 PM | 2 PM | 4 PM | 6 PM | 8 PM | 10 PM | 12 AM | 2 AM | 4 AM | 6 AM |

Major Myth 3: Eating Breakfast Helps You Lose Weight

If cutting calories and exercising are the first and second commandments of weight loss, then eating breakfast has to be the third. Most health experts are convinced that breakfast is the most important meal of the day.

But is it?

Let's start with the typical breakfast foods generally consumed—waffles, cereal, toast, muffins, bagels, doughnuts, and breakfast sandwiches. They are all highly processed grains and *loaded* with sugar. These are some of the absolute *worst* foods you can eat for any meal, let alone breakfast, especially if you want to lose weight.

Is Breakfast Even Necessary?

More and more studies are now showing that the best breakfast may be none at all. Let's look at the evidence.

A 2013 report published in the *American Journal of Clinical Nutrition* found that only a handful of rigorous clinical studies had even *looked* at breakfast's role in weight loss and maintenance.[4] And those studies found either that skipping breakfast had no significant effect on weight gain or that people who partook of a morning meal ended up consuming more calories than people who didn't.

Plenty of less rigorous, observational studies have found an association between eating breakfast and being overweight, but what these studies have *not* found is a direct causal relationship. What that means is that our national obsession with fueling up before starting the day is based on a mere untested assumption.

Skipping Breakfast Can Lead to Weight Loss and Promote Health

Hunger is a basic human drive that can't be easily suppressed, and anyone attempting to start serious calorie restriction is virtually guaranteed to fail over the long term.

Fortunately, recent research suggests that intermittent calorie restriction—short periods of abstaining from foods, known as intermittent fasting, or what I call "effortless eating," appears to provide health benefits similar to those associated with constant calorie restriction.

One of the best things about this way of eating is that

you're *not* supposed to starve yourself. You're not required to restrict the amount of food you eat at all—just choose healthy foods and be careful to minimize carbs and replace them with healthy fats.

And one of the easiest ways to incorporate effortless eating into your life is to create a habit of skipping or delaying breakfast until you are eating all your food in an eight-to-ten-hour window. Avoiding food for long stretches during the day requires enormous discipline, while nighttime fasting doesn't. (After all, it's hard to eat when you're sleeping.) Breakfast also tends to be one of the most solitary meals of the day, the one you typically eat on the run and that you, in terms of socialization or relaxation, enjoy the least.

It will require some willpower and self-discipline to reach this eight-to-ten-hour window because until your body shifts to fat-burning mode, you will still have sugar cravings. However, once you are adapted to burn fat as your primary fuel, you can easily go fourteen to sixteen hours and not be hungry. So now you are not on a "diet" but on an effective lifestyle modification that you can effortlessly follow for the rest of your life because you can cycle between feast and famine modes. (More on this in a moment.)

Omitting breakfast therefore will make it easier for you to control your food cravings and hunger throughout the day. This is an excellent strategy to eliminate cravings for sugar and junk foods.

I remember sharing this secret with a lab assistant in my office. She had gained thirty pounds after she'd had her child seven years earlier. Despite many attempts to lose the weight, she, like so many others, had been unsuccessful.

One day when she was drawing my blood, I asked her if she would ever consider trying my best strategy for losing body fat—this type of intermittent fasting. She agreed and gave it a try.

Within several months, she had lost the thirty pounds. And here is the key: she did it effortlessly, with no cravings and no need for incredible willpower or self-discipline.

Major Myth 4: Eat Several Small Meals Each Day

I suspect you have heard that eating several small meals a day will boost your metabolism. But not only is this strategy impractical and time consuming, it will likely cause you to gain weight rather than lose it. Why? Because it does little to help your body manufacture enough of the needed enzymes to efficiently burn your stored body fat. However, restricting your mealtimes to an eight-to-ten-hour window is a powerful catalyst to help you lose weight, by increasing the production of these fat-burning enzymes. It will also tend to reduce your production of the enzymes that burn sugar, making you better equipped to tap into your fat stores for fuel.

In addition, your body is not designed to regularly and consistently digest food all day long. In fact, your body is adapted to function during regular periods of no food. Your ancestors rarely had access to food 24/7 as you do today, and your genes, metabolism, and biochemistry are likely optimized for the more sporadic, intermittent meals that they ate. They regularly cycled through periods of feasts and famine. As a result, the human body has evolved to store fat to help people survive periods of famine. The problem is that you are probably always in feasting mode, eating three meals if not more every day, and rarely undergo regular periods of fasting.

What the media calls "intermittent fasting" and I call "effortless eating" today is what our ancestors knew as a regular way of life. During periods of fasting—which are practiced in every major religion—they burned their body fat for fuel. You too have this ability but have likely trained your body not to use it. Just as with building muscle, the ability to burn body fat is "use it or lose it." If you don't regularly challenge your fat-burning enzymes to burn fat, they will tend to ratchet down to nonfunction mode over time. If you do exercise them, they will regain and retain the ability to effortlessly burn fat as a fuel in times of famine.

The good news is that when you skip breakfast, you mimic the natural fluctuations in food availability that your ancestors encountered and stimulate your body's famine mode. If you have been feasting for many years or even decades, it will take a while for you to improve your insulin and leptin resistance, during which time you'll want to stick to a scheduled plan of effortless eating during an eight-to-ten-hour window each day.

Once you are no longer overweight and have normal blood pressure, blood sugar, and cholesterol ratios, then you can start effortlessly feasting again, so long as you choose healthy foods. If these bellwethers of health start to climb higher, you will likely benefit from stopping the feast mode long enough to normalize your weight or body fat. You merely need to listen to what your body is telling you and adjust your food pattern to how you are feeling and to what symptoms you are experiencing. In this way, you can cycle back and forth between feast and famine just as your ancestors did.

Powerful Benefits of Effortless Eating

Training your body to burn fat for fuel and eating only during an eight-to-ten-hour window creates the conditions your body needs to function optimally and to repair itself and ward off diseases effortlessly. This is the most powerful benefit of effortless eating.

Here are more specific ways this approach to healing empowers your body:

Reduces Cravings for Sugar and Other Unhealthy Foods

Aside from turning you into an efficient fat-burning machine, effortless eating can remove your cravings for sugar and snack foods, thereby making it virtually effortless to maintain a healthy body weight.

Promotes Human Growth Hormone (HGH)

One of the mechanisms that makes fasting so effective as a weight-loss tool is that it provokes the secretion of human growth hormone (HGH). If you're over the age of thirty, especially if you lead an increasingly sedentary lifestyle, you've likely entered a phase known as somatopause (age-related growth hormone deficiency).

HGH, commonly referred to as the "fitness hormone," is something you want to encourage, as it serves an important role in maintaining health, fitness, and longevity. It also promotes muscle growth and revs up your metabolism—meaning it helps you lose weight without sacrificing muscle mass.

The only other strategy that can compete, in terms of dramatically boosting HGH levels, is high-intensity interval training. (More on this in Healing Principle 4.)

Normalizes Hunger Levels

Fasting inhibits the release of ghrelin, which is known as the "hunger hormone," thereby helping to normalize or reduce your appetite.

Boosts Your Brain Health

Burning fat as your body's primary fuel will boost production of a protein called brain-derived neurotrophic factor (BDNF). BDNF activates brain stem cells to convert into new nerve cells. It triggers many other chemicals that catalyze healing events. And it protects brain cells from changes associated with Alzheimer's and Parkinson's diseases.

BDNF expresses itself in nerves and muscles, where it protects them from degradation. It is produced during high-intensity exercise, so if you combine fasting with these exercises, you will obtain a powerful synergy to increase this valuable brain-building and brain-repairing hormone.

BDNF is actively involved in both your muscles *and* your brain. That cross-connection helps explain why a physical workout can have such a beneficial impact on your brain tissue—and why the combination of intermittent fasting with high-intensity exercise appears to be a particularly potent health-boosting combination.

Dramatically Lowers Your Risk of Cardiovascular Disease

Recent studies have found compelling links between fasting and reduced risk of heart disease.[5] A 2012 study with a large percentage of Mormon participants (who are encouraged to fast one day a month) found that those who fasted regularly had a 58 percent lower risk of heart disease compared with those who never fasted.[6] While the study didn't establish the cause of the reduction in risk, a few benefits of intermittent fasting do work to promote cardiovascular health, including:

- Moderating levels of dangerous visceral (or belly) fat, which is associated with a higher risk of cardiovascular disease

- Lowering inflammation
- Reproducing some of the heart benefits associated with physical exercise
- Lowering triglyceride levels

Helps Treat or Prevent Cancer and Inhibits the Aging Process

Compelling new research suggests that if you have insulin or leptin resistance, lowering that resistance can reduce your risk of cancer[7] or help treat a cancer you might have.[8]

Fasting inhibits your mTOR pathway, which many experts believe plays an important role in driving the aging process, as it accelerates cell proliferation. You probably never heard of mTOR, but it is an ancient biochemical pathway that scientists discovered only recently, when they were researching how a cancer drug, rapamycin, worked. The name mTOR is actually derived from that cancer drug: Mammalian Target Of Rapamycin. By inhibiting the mTOR pathway, effortless eating slows down the rate of growth—and thus aging—of cells, thereby promoting longevity and overall health.

Effortless eating also encourages longevity by decreasing the accumulation of oxidative radicals in cells, thereby preventing oxidative damage to cellular proteins, lipids, and nucleic acids associated with aging and disease. Fasting induces a cellular stress response (similar to that induced by exercise) in which cells upregulate the expression of genes that increase the capacity to cope with stress and resist disease and aging.

Improves Gut Bacteria

When you incorporate effortless eating into your life regularly, another phenomenal side effect will occur: it will radically improve the beneficial bacteria in your gut, which play an enormous role in how healthy you are.

Supporting healthy gut bacteria is one of the most important actions you can take to improve your immune system (see Healing Principle 6). It radically reduces your risk of getting coughs, colds, flus, and other infections. You will sleep better, have more energy, enjoy increased mental clarity, and concentrate better. Essentially every aspect of your health will improve as your gut flora becomes balanced.

How to Shift to Effortless Eating

E ffortless eating is one of the most effective ways I know of to shed excess weight and repair the metabolic dysfunction that leads to so many of the chronic diseases that are pillaging your health. Once you've adapted to burning fat, you'll typically find that your sugar cravings will vanish without a trace.

Start Slowly

The last thing you want to do, however, is jump right into full-blown intermittent fasting. You want to allow your body to adapt gradually to burning fat as its primary fuel. If you are only mildly insulin and leptin resistant, the process could take just a few weeks. If you have major insulin or leptin resistance, however, it could take up to a few months.

Start by not eating anything for three hours before you go to bed. If you sleep for 7 or 8 hours, then you already have 10 to 11 hours under your belt. You need to go only another 3 to 6 hours before your next meal. But this is something you will work up to over a few weeks—you won't start the program at this level.

At first, just go as long as you comfortably can without eating breakfast. Note the time, and gradually extend that time later each day, to the point where your first meal of the day is 14 to 16 hours after your last meal.

When you start skipping breakfast, you will probably feel hungry and even experience a lack of energy. I assure you—this will pass. This is the only time where effortless eating isn't so effortless, and you need to use some self-discipline and willpower. But if you hang in there, trust me—your hunger and cravings for sugar and junk food will disappear, and you will find it very easy to eat this way. Once your body adjusts, it will truly be effortless, as you won't be hungry. Many times you won't even remember that you haven't eaten.

In the hours that you do eat, minimize carbs like pasta, bread, and potatoes and exchange them for healthy green leafy vegetables and healthy fats like butter, eggs, avocado, coconut oil, olive oil, and nuts like macadamia and pecans because they are lower in protein. Please keep in mind that proper nutrition becomes even *more* important when fasting, so addressing your food choices really should be your first step.

Sources of High-Quality Fats

- Olives and olive oil
- Coconuts and coconut oil
- Butter made from raw pasture-fed organic milk
- Raw nuts, especially those low in protein, such as macadamias and pecans
- Organic pastured egg. The less you cook them, the better, as many nutrients in yolks are susceptible to heat damage. Soft-boiled and poached are your best options.
- Avocados

Once you wake up your fat-burning enzymes, you will not be dependent on finding a quick source of sugar to fuel your glycogen stores. You will no longer have to rely on an ever-replenished supply of fast-burning carbs for fuel and will be able to finally burn your stored fat as fuel.

During the transition to burning fat, you will likely have sugar cravings and may even experience a lack of energy. If that happens, that would be a signal to use some coconut oil as a source of energy. Mix one tablespoon of coconut oil with one tablespoon of raw almond butter and spread the mixture on celery sticks for a snack. Or blend it into a glass of kefir or fresh green vegetable juice. Stir a tablespoon into the soup you have for lunch. Coconut oil will not add to your glycogen stores, and its many short-chained fats are easily digested, to provide you with fuel very similar to sugar. You can even eat it during the time you are fasting.

If you develop any hypoglycemic tendencies, such as headaches, weakness, tremors, or irritability, you can address them by using coconut oil. Hypoglycemia can get increasingly dangerous the longer you go without eating to level out your blood sugar.

The Cravings Will Pass

Always listen to your body, and go slowly. Shifting to fat-burning mode typically takes several weeks, though it can take longer. But once you make the shift, what happens to your cravings for sweets and junk food will be nothing short of magical. Effortless eating rapidly normalizes your appetite and radically decreases your desire for sweets and junk food.

Remember, it will take a few weeks and some initial discipline, and you have to do it gradually. But once you successfully switch to fat-burning mode, you'll be easily able to fast effortlessly for sixteen hours and not feel hungry. Once you retrain your body not to expect food all day every day or immediately after you wake up, maintaining your new trim physique will truly feel effortless.

Other Tips

Skip dinner instead of breakfast. Most people find that skipping breakfast is the easiest and most practical approach. But for whatever reason, you may find that skipping dinner is better. That's fine. The important principle is to restrict your food intake to an eight-to-ten-hour window, to stimulate your fat-burning enzymes.

Relax. Remember to relax and not sweat the details. Trust that your body will adapt to this new style of eating. It isn't a permanent lifestyle change, if losing weight is your aim—just a matter of a few weeks or months, which will pass. Even if you are at a healthy weight, you'll likely benefit from undergoing regular cycles of feast and famine to retain the ability to effortlessly burn fat and resist the chronic diseases that are currently plaguing our society.

Stay busy. If you're just sitting around thinking about how hungry you are, you'll be far more likely to struggle with implementing the shift than if you stay busy.

Who Shouldn't Fast?

If you're pregnant or breastfeeding, you're better off avoiding any type of fasting or timed meal schedule until you've normalized your blood glucose and insulin levels, or weaned the baby.

People living with chronic excessive stress that results in severe adrenal exhaustion should also avoid fasting. Wait to adopt effortless eating until the time of stress and/or adrenal fatigue has passed.

ENLIST THE COLD

Another way to nudge your body to burn more fat is to expose it to cold temperatures. Drinking ice cold water, immersing your lower body in the coldest water you can stand (too cold or too much of your body, and you may go into shock—use your tolerance as a guide and don't overdo it!), and working or exercising outdoors in winter all fit the bill. Cold exposure triggers your brown fat—the type of fat that burns calories in order to generate heat. This benefit of exposing yourself to cold temperatures is all the more reason to get yourself out of the house for an outdoor workout in the winter, or to join in the New Year's Day tradition of swimming in the ocean.

| ADVANCED EFFORTLESS HEALING |

Exercise While Fasting

Although effortless eating offers a host of benefits on its own, a simple way to amplify them even further is to exercise while you're in the fasted state.

Here's how it works: your body's fat-burning processes are controlled by your sympathetic nervous system (SNS), and your SNS is activated by both exercise and a lack of food.

Eating a full meal, particularly carbohydrates, before your workout inhibits your SNS and reduces the fat-burning effects of your exercise. Eating lots of carbs also activates your parasympathetic nervous system (PNS), which promotes energy storage—the opposite of what you're aiming for.

On the other hand, the combination of fasting and exercising essentially forces your body to shed fat.

You will likely want to avoid working out while fasting initially. But working out in a fasted state is effective because your body has a preservation mechanism that protects your active muscle from wasting itself. So if you don't have sufficient fuel in your system when you exercise, you're going to break down other tissues *but not the active muscle*—that is, the muscle being exercised.

On the days that you work out while fasting, you should eat a recovery meal thirty minutes after your workout. That will limit any muscle loss and damage to tissues from your workout. Fast-assimilating, high-quality whey protein is ideal.

Once you are fat-adapted, you can cycle between feast and famine modes. Try eating healthy fresh fruits (not juices) before you exercise—your body will use the sugar as fuel and not store it as fat. That will eliminate some of the problems with excess fructose and yet allow you to reap the biological benefit and joy of eating fresh fruit.

> **Putting the benefits of effortless eating to work for you can be as simple as skipping breakfast and exercising first thing in the morning, when your stomach is empty.**

Your Effortless Action Plan

1. Eat more healthy fats and as few sugars and grains as possible.

2. Stop eating and drinking at least three hours before you go to bed.

3. Delay your first meal of the day as long as you can—work up to at least noon.

4. Restrict consuming calories to an eight-to-ten-hour window.

5. Exercise while fasting to improve muscle regeneration and repair.

6. Once you are fat-adapted, you can cycle between feast and famine modes.

HEALERS	HURTERS
✓ Organic, pastured eggs	✗ Rice
✓ Avocados	✗ Pasta
✓ Coconut oil	✗ Bread
✓ Most raw nuts, especially macadamias and pecans	✗ Sugars
✓ Olives and olive oil	✗ Agave
✓ Raw pastured dairy	✗ Honey
✓ Skipping breakfast, eating dinner early, and no late-night snacking	✗ Eating frequent meals throughout the day
✓ Exercising first thing in the morning, before eating	✗ Carb-loading before a workout

TIME TAKEN, TIME SAVED

Skipping one or two meals a day will easily free up a load of time that you can repurpose to other items that you just never seem to get to. It can easily save you hours every week.

Switching to burning fat as your primary fuel can take anywhere from a few weeks to a few months. Once you do it, though, you will have enormous freedom. You won't have to rely on eating junk food to prevent your blood sugar from crashing. That will just make you feel sluggish and tired, because you have taught your body how to effortlessly burn fat again. It will be able to burn fat for your next meal. So rather than rely on some unhealthy junk food, you will be able to delay your eating until you have access to healthy food.

Healing Principle 4

Exercise Less and Gain More Benefits

At a Glance

✓ Your health, mobility, and freedom from pain in older age depend on your dedication to moving frequently and wisely.

✓ Reducing the length of time you sit each day is even more important than getting regular exercise.

✓ Addressing poor posture is a useful strategy to optimize your health.

✓ Traditional cardio exercises are highly inefficient and can be radically improved.

✓ Short bursts of high-intensity interval exercise several times a week offer powerful rewards that conventional cardio doesn't.

✓ Strength training and stretching round out a comprehensive fitness plan.

For too many years, I made the mistake of ignoring the dangers of poor posture while sitting, and sitting too long. Within the past few years, a number of studies have shown that even if you are very fit and work out at the gym five to seven days a week, or are an elite athlete, sitting for most of your day will put you at much higher risk of dying prematurely.[1]

I admit, at first I simply did not believe these studies. But the evidence has accumulated to the point that I am now firmly convinced that you will increase your risk of premature death if you sit all day.

While formal exercise is a crucial component of Effortless Healing (more on this in a moment), you simply cannot expect to enjoy optimal wellness if you work out a few times a week but spend most of the rest of your days sitting.

I know what you're probably thinking: How does this jibe with my job?

I'm happy to report that you can still keep your office job and remain healthy. I sit at a computer up to twelve hours a day, for example. You simply have to incorporate the types of movements and postural adjustments that I learned from a top NASA expert, a world-renowned researcher at the Mayo Clinic, and a leading posture expert.

Intermittent Movement: Lessen the Damage from Sitting

Going to the gym a few times a week for an hour simply isn't going to counteract hours upon hours of uninterrupted sitting. That's why getting hung up on a once-a-day exercise routine is putting the cart before the horse. First you need to make sure you're consciously increasing your nonexercise movements during your day. Once you develop a habit of doing nonexercise activities, you can add structured exercise.

Dr. Joan Vernikos, former director of NASA's Life Sciences Division, was a scientist with NASA for thirty years. She was responsible for addressing the damage that the microgravity of space was causing the astronauts. In her research, she learned that excessive sitting mimics the microgravity environment of space and has many of the same negative health results. "We are not designed to sit continuously. We are designed to squat. We are designed to kneel. Sitting is okay, but uninterrupted sitting is bad for us," Dr. Vernikos says. Her book *Sitting Kills, Moving Heals* presents a simple yet powerful scientific explanation for why sitting has such a dramatic impact on health, and it provides ways to simply and easily counteract the ill effects of sitting.

Even though I had performed structured exercises for over forty years, I was guilty of sitting down a vast majority of the rest of the day. Although I was physiologically very fit, my musculoskeletal health was suffering, as I was experiencing a lot of daily aches and stiffness and loads of low back pain. In fact, I couldn't stand or walk for long periods without pain. So I was drawn to her book.

Dr. Vernikos's discovery was as revolutionary as it was counterintuitive. She found that frequently interrupting your sitting by merely standing up can eliminate most of the negative side effects of excessive sitting. You need to do this about thirty-five times a day, which for most people means standing up about every fifteen minutes. It doesn't get more effortless than that.

You can easily find a timer on the Internet to download for free. But many of them have an alarm sound that can easily startle you and potentially disrupt your adrenals (because of the stress) if you listen to it all day long. There are several options to remind you to move every fifteen minutes, from free apps on your phone to a fitness band that gently vibrates to remind you to move after inactivity. Find something you like, and use it.

Dr. Vernikos found out that the act of standing in and of

itself isn't what benefits health; it's actually *the change in posture* that is the most powerful signal. That's why standing desks are not much better than sitting ones. Your body was designed to function best when you treat it and feed it as our ancient ancestors did. None of them had desk jobs where they sat most of the day. So if you are like me and have a desk job, it will be really important for you to take proactive steps to prevent the inevitable damage that occurs from simply doing your job. There's no other way to put it: too much sitting abuses your body.

The good news is that you don't need to spend hours moving each day. The key is to frequently interrupt your sitting—it's as simple as remembering to stand up. Going from a sitting position to a standing position changes your body's relationship to gravity, and that's what stimulates your muscles to stay strong, your circulation to keep moving, and your overall physiology to remain responsive. In addition, frequently *moving and shifting position* when you're sitting down will also reap the benefits of changing your relationship to gravity.

> **A good rule of thumb for making sure you don't sit too long is to stand up every fifteen minutes or so.**

| ADVANCED EFFORTLESS HEALING |
Stand Up and Move

If you're already in good shape, then you may want to add a bit more of an exercise challenge to your day, beyond merely standing up. You can interrupt your sitting every fifteen minutes to do any of dozens of healthy movements for thirty seconds or so to get your blood flowing. The options are virtually limitless. I have over thirty videos of short exercises you can do on my website (at http://fitness.mercola.com/sites/fitness/archive/2014/04/11/intermittent-movement.aspx). It's best to mix them up so that you interrupt your sitting with a wide variety of different movements.

Dr. James Levine is an esteemed professor and obesity researcher at the Mayo Clinic and is one of the leading advocates for this approach. He states that there are now over 10,000 studies documenting the importance of interrupting the average eight hours a day most of us sit. One of the best and simplest options, though, might be using a stand-up desk. If this isn't feasible for you, try to walk for ten minutes for every hour that you are sitting. The walking should be done every hour, not all at once. Fitness trackers are an emerging new product, and by 2020, experts predict the market will be ten times larger than it is now. These trackers can be used to calculate your daily steps, and even how long you are sleeping.

Pay Attention to Posture

Posture is at the crossroads of many different spheres of health—circulatory, respiratory, digestive, reproductive, and musculoskeletal. The way you sit, stand, and move affects the way you interact with gravity.

By understanding the functional biomechanics of your body and working with gravity instead of against it, you will radically decrease the normal pains of aging. You will be supple and pain free as you age, and able to participate more fully in life.

My eyes were opened to the power of posture by Dr. Eric Goodman, who was trained as a chiropractor and developed a series of exercises called Foundation Training that effectively eliminates most back pain.

While conventional advice tells you to tuck in your pelvis to maintain an S-shaped spine, this is not natural. Rather, having your back straight, your lumbar area relatively flat, and your buttocks protruding slightly is a far better posture. This is the natural stance of toddlers and most traditional cultures.

Ideally you want to *antevert* your pelvis—in other words, rotate the top of your hip forward and down. This is easy if you imagine you have a tail. Don't rotate the top of your hipbone backward—that would put your tail between your legs. The better position is to put your tail behind you. Using that visual picture will make it easier for you to figure out in which direction to move your pelvis.

When you tuck your pelvis backward (or *retrovert* it), you lose about a third of the volume in your pelvic cavity, which compresses your internal organs. Primal posture, on the other hand, provides an ideal architecture for your lungs to move freely and allows your digestive and reproductive organs enough space to function optimally.

Once you have your pelvis properly tilted, while you are sitting it is crucial to make sure your shoulders are properly positioned. You can achieve this by simply rolling one shoulder at a time backward.

Understanding gravity as a force and adjusting your posture accordingly also promotes bone health. Your bones have evolved to retain calcium as a response to being triggered by gravity. When your bones line up properly, tiny electrical forces are generated that cue calcium to stay in your bones instead of going off into the bloodstream. If your bones are improperly aligned as you go through your day, these electrical forces are absent. As a result, your bones become weak and more predisposed to breaking. Bone density is truly a "use it [properly] or lose it" proposition.

There's simply no doubt about it—to have a well-functioning body, you must learn how to optimize your posture.

Formal Exercise

While intermittent movement and good posture are crucial pieces of the Effortless Healing equation, for optimal wellness you also need to include formal exercise.

Benefits of Formal Exercise

The primary reason is that regular exercise helps normalize your glucose, insulin, and leptin levels,[2] which, as I've mentioned, is the single most important improvement you can make in your quest to prevent and treat chronic disease. Regular exercise will help your insulin and leptin receptors work more effectively.

Exercise benefits other systems of your body as well—both directly and indirectly:

Muscles   When you exercise, you increase your breathing and heart rate. That sends more blood and oxygen to your muscles, which strengthens and energizes them. Also, as you work your muscles, you create tiny tears in them that are then rebuilt bigger and stronger during the healing process. More exercise equals more muscle.

Lungs   As your muscles call for more oxygen (as much as fifteen times more oxygen than when you're at rest), your breathing rate increases. Once the muscles surrounding your lungs cannot move any faster, you've reached what's called your VO2 max—your maximum capacity of oxygen use. As you continue to exercise over time, your VO2 max will get higher, meaning your breathing will be more efficient at all times.

Heart   With physical activity, as I've mentioned, your heart rate increases to supply more oxygenated blood to your muscles. The more times you exercise, the more efficiently your heart will be able to work. As a side effect, this increased efficiency will also reduce your *resting* heart rate, meaning your heart will have to work less hard to do its job of circulating your blood even when you're *not* exercising. Over time you'll also trigger the creation of new blood vessels, which will lower your blood pressure.

Brain   The increased blood flow also benefits your brain, allowing it to almost immediately function better. That's why you tend to feel more focused after a workout. Furthermore, exercising regularly will promote the growth of new brain cells, which can help boost memory and learning.

A number of neurotransmitters are also triggered, such as endorphins, serotonin, dopamine, glutamate, and GABA. Some of these are well known for their role in mood control. Exercise, in fact, is one of the most effective prevention and treatment strategies for depression.

Joints and Bones   Peak bone mass is achieved in adulthood, then begins a slow decline. But exercise can help you to maintain healthy bone mass as you get older. It can place as much as five or six times more than your body weight on your bones; in response to that stress, they are cued to get stronger.

In fact, weight-bearing exercise is actually one of the most effective ways of preventing osteoporosis. Without it, your bones can easily become porous and soft and hence more brittle.

Less Exercise Equals More

If you're like most people, one of the biggest hurdles in maintaining an exercise program is finding the time to do it on a regular basis. The great news is that you may never again have to resort to this excuse. Exercise by definition isn't effortless, but with the new insights I'm about to share, you can effortlessly fit it into your schedule. You'll be able to dramatically improve your fitness levels and markers of health in only minutes of exercise effort each week.

> **An increasing body of evidence supports the notion that you can cut your workout time significantly while reaping greater benefits.**

Yes, I said "minutes."

This "get more in less time" approach to fitness suits my goal for readers of this book: to offer simple, effective, efficient ways for you to help your body run at its maximum, with as little effort—and interference—on your part as possible. If it sounds too good to be true, I completely understand. For forty years, I was fooled, too. During those four decades, I ran tens of thousands of miles and wasted thousands of hours in an effort to exercise properly doing traditional cardio.

I have come to believe that while cardio is certainly useful, there are far better ways to improve health through exercise. Spending long periods of time running, jogging, walking, or doing cardio machines at the gym is relatively inefficient; it simply doesn't provide enough benefit to compensate for the time invested.

Peak Fitness: A Prescription for Vitality

Walk into any gym, and you'll see most of the people crowding around the cardio equipment. But there's actually a way to exercise that's *far* more effective than walking or running on a treadmill or using an elliptical machine for an hour. It's called Peak Fitness.

Peak Fitness is a term I coined for a technique I learned from Phil Campbell. Phil helped me understand that by not doing high-intensity exercises, I was leaving a lot of benefits on the table. Peak Fitness takes only twenty minutes. (If you graph your heart

IF JEFF CAN EXERCISE, WHAT'S YOUR EXCUSE?

Over the course of my career, I have treated more than 25,000 patients—but one in particular made a significant impact on me. Jeff was a thirty-nine-year-old man with a rare condition called Cushing's disease. His pituitary gland was making too many adrenal-stimulating hormones, and he would have died from too much cortisol if not treated.

Before he came to me, he had gone to the University of Chicago to surgically excise a pituitary tumor. Unfortunately an anesthesiology complication arose during the surgery, and as a result he was paralyzed from the waist down and had no use of his legs.

The misfortune didn't stop there. The surgeons accidentally clipped his optic nerve, which also left him blind.

This was an obvious tragedy. But what impressed me most about Jeff was that although he was blind and paralyzed from the waist down, he was exercising regularly with his upper body while in his wheelchair. He fully embraced the value of exercise.

The take-home message for me is that if Jeff could find a way to exercise, then so can anyone, especially using the twenty-first-century insights revealed in this chapter.

rate during that twenty minutes, you'll see that it peaks eight times). And of those twenty, *you are only exercising hard for **four minutes***. But those four minutes are *really* intense.

Most people who adopt Peak Fitness notice the following benefits within a few weeks:

- Lower body fat
- Dramatically improved muscle tone
- Firmer skin and reduced wrinkles
- Boosted energy and sexual desire
- Improved athletic speed and performance
- Fitness goals achieved much faster

But these aren't even the most powerful benefits. Peak Fitness exercises can improve your insulin sensitivity by nearly 25 percent with a time investment of less than *a few hours a month.* That is, you can significantly improve your health without having to eliminate from your calendar many dozens of hours of other commitments.

Remember, normalizing your insulin level is the most important factor in optimizing your overall health and helping to prevent disease of all kinds, from diabetes to heart disease to cancer and everything in between.

Peak Fitness Boosts Growth Hormone

Human growth hormone (HGH) is essential for optimal health, strength, and vigor. It has been shown to significantly improve insulin sensitivity, boost fat loss, and increase muscle growth.

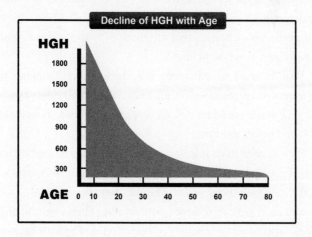

As you reach your thirties and beyond, you enter somatopause, and your levels of HGH drop off quite dramatically (see the graph). This is part of what drives the aging process. If you are over thirty, you likely have low levels of this important hormone. But by using Peak Fitness exercises you can return your levels close to where they were in your twenties.

The longer you can keep your body producing healthy levels of HGH, the longer you will experience robust health and strength. HGH is so effective at increasing muscle mass that many competitive and professional athletes spend a thousand dollars a month to inject it; they chance being barred from their sport and run an increased risk of cancer. Fortunately, you don't have to spend money or gamble with your health to get those benefits. High-intensity interval-type training will give a natural and significant boost to your HGH production. And when your body produces it naturally, feedback loops will prevent you from overdosing so there is no increased risk of cancer.

In addition to increasing HGH production, Peak Fitness also boosts the hormone called brain-derived neurotrophic factor (BDNF). As I discussed on page 97, this important hormone keeps your brain young, sharp, and actively engaged by converting brain stem cells into new nerve cells. It also protects your brain cells from changes that are involved with the development of Parkinson's and Alzheimer's.

Peak Fitness's benefits don't stop there. Other hormones that are improved are testosterone, adiponectin, glucagon-like peptide-1 (GLP-1), cholecystokinin (CCK), and melanocortins, as well as insulin and leptin resistance.

All you need to do is look at nature for clues as to what an ideal type of exercise might be. Children and most animals in the wild do not run marathons or lift weights; they move at high speeds for very short periods of time and then rest. This is natural and, I believe, optimizes their health and production of growth hormone.

> In twenty minutes or less, including your warm-up and cool-down, Peak Fitness provides more benefits than an hour-long cardio workout.

Increasing Muscle Mass

Peak Fitness benefits your muscles in ways that other forms of exercise simply can't. So you can fully appreciate this advantage, let me give you a little background on how muscles work.

Your body has three types of muscle fibers:

- **Slow twitch.** These red muscle fibers are filled with loads of capillaries and mitochondria and hence a lot of oxygen (which is why they are red). Traditionally performed cardio and strength training work *only* your slow muscle fibers.
- **Fast twitch.** These white fibers oxygenate quickly but are five times faster than the slow fibers. Power training, or plyometric-type bursts of exercise, will engage these fast muscle fibers.
- **Superfast twitch.** These white muscle fibers contain far less blood and less densely packed mitochondria. They are what you use when you do anaerobic, short-burst exercises like sprinting on an elliptical machine, pushing a weighted sled, or climbing stairs. Imagine your cat or dog at play: it runs for short fast bursts, rests, and then repeats. High-intensity cardio is the form of exercise that will engage these superfast fibers. They're ten times faster than slow fibers, and *they are the key to producing growth hormone!*

Currently, the vast majority of people who exercise, including many athletes such as marathon runners, train by primarily using their slow muscle fibers. That has the unfortunate effect of causing the superfast fibers to decrease or atrophy.

Getting maximum cardiovascular benefit requires working all three types of muscle fiber and their associated energy systems. That simply *can't* be done with traditional cardio, which activates *only* slow twitch muscles. If your fitness routine doesn't work your white muscle, you aren't really working your heart in the most beneficial way. That's because your heart has two different metabolic processes:

- The aerobic, which requires oxygen for fuel; and
- The anaerobic, which requires no oxygen.

Traditional strength training and cardio exercises work only the aerobic process, but high-intensity interval exercises work both your aerobic *and* your anaerobic processes, which is what you need for optimal cardiovascular benefit. This is why with traditional cardio, you may not see the results you desire, even when you're spending an hour on the treadmill several times a week.

While your heart is designed to work very hard and will be strengthened from doing so, it's designed to do so only *intermittently* and for short periods—not for an hour or more at a time. So contrary to popular belief, extended extreme cardio sets in motion inflammatory mechanisms that can actually *damage* your heart.

Peak Fitness Workout

You can start a Peak Fitness program with any type of exercise. While having access to a gym or exercise equipment will give you a larger variety of options, it's not necessary. You can easily perform the exercises with something as simple as running.

Your goal is to get your heart rate up to its calculated maximum, which is 220 minus your age. That's where the "magic" happens that will trigger your growth hormone release.

If you are using exercise equipment, I recommend that you start off with a recumbent bicycle and then progress to my favorite, the elliptical machine. Be careful about using a treadmill, as it will be slower to respond to speed changes and easier for you to fall off when you're tired. Sprinting is ideal, but if you aren't careful, you can sprain your hamstrings or pull a muscle. So be very careful about stretching properly, paying careful attention to your hamstrings prior to sprinting.

Here are the core principles:

- Warm up for three minutes.
- Exercise as hard and fast as you can for 30 seconds. You should feel like you couldn't possibly go on another few seconds.
- Recover for 90 seconds, still moving, but at a much slower pace.
- Repeat the high-intensity exercise-and-recovery cycle seven more times. (When you're first starting out, you may be able to do only *two or three* repetitions of the high-intensity intervals. As you get fitter, just keep adding repetitions until you're doing eight during your 20-minute session.)
- Afterward, cool down for two minutes by slowing the pace of the exercise you were doing during these "sprints." After you've cooled down, your total time working out will be 21 minutes (less if you don't complete all eight reps of the high-intensity-rest cycle).
- It may take you a few weeks to a few months to work up to eight reps.

At the end of each 30-second high-intensity interval, you will want to reach these markers:

- It will be relatively hard to breathe and nearly impossible to talk because you are in oxygen debt.
- You will sweat. Typically this begins in the second or third repetition, unless you have a thyroid issue and don't sweat much normally.
- Your body temperature will rise.
- Lactic acid will increase, and you will feel a muscle "burn."

This marker will disappear as you become fitter, but the first three will persist.

Perform this workout two or three times a week. Doing it more frequently can be counterproductive, as your body needs recovery. If you feel the urge to do more, make sure you're really pushing yourself *as hard as you can* during those two-or-three-times-per-week sessions, rather than increasing the frequency. Intensity is *key* for reaping all the benefits that interval training can offer.

If you have a history of heart disease or any medical concern, please be sure to get clearance from your health care professional before you start. There are some uncommon conditions where high-intensity exercises are best avoided.

Add Variety

Doing the Peak Fitness workout two or three times a week is the core of your program. That will get you more fit than most of the population. However, to truly keep your body strong, flexible, and pain free, you should incorporate a couple other elements, including:

Strength Training Strength training (also known as weight-bearing exercise or resistance training) improves many areas of health: it is one of the most effective remedies against osteoporosis. It has been found to have a beneficial impact on gene expression—it not only slows aging in seniors but actually returns their gene expression to youthful levels. It's also very beneficial for glucose control and cardiovascular health. Gaining more muscle through strength training helps people lose excess fat and helps prevent age-related muscle loss.

To ensure that you're optimizing the benefits of your Peak

Fitness program, round it out with a strength training routine, performed one to three times per week. You need to do enough repetitions to exhaust your muscles, so use a weight that's heavy enough to exhaust your muscles in fewer than twelve repetitions, yet light enough that you can do a minimum of four repetitions. It is important *not* to exercise the same muscle groups every day. Muscles typically need two days of rest to recover, repair, and rebuild.

Stretching Your body was designed to move, so when you sit all day long, it gradually stiffens up and loses its full range of motion. Being sedentary leaves you inflexible and susceptible to pain, especially low back pain. Even when you interrupt your sitting with frequent standing breaks, your muscles and joints still have to be put through their full ranges of motion in order to stay supple and strong. So stretching plays a vital supporting role in your Effortless Healing plan.

My favorite type of stretching is dynamic stretching, in which you hold each stretch for only two seconds while actively using your muscles to move in the direction of the stretch. For example, you lie flat on your back and raise one leg straight up into the air. You use your quadriceps muscles (on the front of the thigh) to move your leg closer to your head, thereby stretching your hamstring muscles (on the back of your thigh).

This form of stretching (known as Active Isolated Stretching, or AIS) works with your body's natural physiological makeup to improve circulation and increase the elasticity of muscle joints—which then aids your body in its continuous quest to repair itself. It also prepares your body for daily activity, counteracting the stiffness that so many wake up with each day. It's an amazing way to get flexibility back into your system, and it's very different from traditional stretching. Perhaps best of all, it takes only minutes to stretch all the major muscle groups of the body.

A gadget that can be immensely helpful in increasing flexibility is the Power Plate—a mechanical platform that moves a few centimeters in three dimensions anywhere from 20 to 40 times a second. These movements increase the force of gravity. Since muscles respond to the forces you place upon them, performing stretches on the Power Plate results in a bigger increase in flexibility than simply performing stretches on the ground.

KEEP YOGA IN MIND

Yoga is a useful discipline that integrates stretching and offers a wide variety of other health benefits as well.

Duke University researchers recently reviewed more than one hundred studies of the effect of yoga on mental health. The lead author, Dr. P. Murali Doraiswamy, a professor of psychiatry and medicine at Duke University Medical Center, told *Time* magazine:

> *Most individuals already know that yoga produces some kind of a calming effect. Individually, people feel better after doing the physical exercise. Mentally, people feel calmer, sharper, maybe more content. We thought it's time to see if we could pull all [the literature] together . . . to see if there's enough evidence that the benefits individual people notice can be used to help people with mental illness.*[3]

According to their findings, yoga appears to have a positive effect on:

- Mild depression
- Sleep problems
- Schizophrenia (among patients using medication)
- ADHD (among patients using medication)

Some of the studies suggest that yoga can have a similar effect to antidepressants and psychotherapy, by influencing neurotransmitters and boosting serotonin. Yoga has also been found to reduce levels of inflammation, oxidative stress, blood lipids, and growth factors.

There's No Time Like the Present!

No matter where you are now on the fitness spectrum, you can start there and reap enormous benefits for your health. If you've been sedentary for any length of time or you're out of shape for some other reason, it's vitally important to get started on using your body better, through regular movement, proper posture, and an intelligent exercise program.

One of the main reasons people don't stick with a workout program is that they go too hard, too fast, and wind up with an injury, illness, or simple exhaustion. So just start small and slow and build up gradually until all elements are included. Be patient with yourself.

Please don't use your age as an excuse. It's never too late to take control of your health, and movement, posture, and exercise are crucial components of well-being at any age.

If you happen to be over forty, though, it's especially important to either start or step up your movement program. Your physical strength, stamina, balance, and flexibility have all started to decline. But everything I outlined in this chapter can help counteract that.

My mom didn't start working out until she was seventy-four and now, at the age of eighty, she has gained significant improvement in strength, range of motion, balance, bone density, and mental clarity.

Whether you're eighteen or eighty, I guarantee that a regular, thoughtful movement routine will make a major difference in your energy level and probably your entire outlook on life. It is really that powerful!

Your Effortless Action Plan

1. Upgrade your exercise regimen by ditching regular cardio and shift to two or three sessions a week of high-intensity interval training. This is basically one hour a week of exercise, spread out over two or three days.

2. At least once a week and as many as three times a week, do a few sets of strength training exercises before or after your Peak Fitness workout, to keep the number of days you work out each week at two or three.

3. Stretch multiple times per week—at least three and as many as seven. Incorporating a ten-minute stretch session into your morning or bedtime routine is a great way to make sure you do it even on the days when you don't work out.

4. If you have a desk job, try to stand up every fifteen minutes to counteract the negative effects of excessive sitting.

5. Pay careful attention to your posture. Learn how to sit, stand, and walk with gravity working for you instead of against you.

HEALERS	HURTERS
✓ Interrupting your sitting every 15 minutes or so by standing or changing position	✗ Sitting for extended stretches of time each day, even if you work out several hours a week
✓ Allowing the tailbone to stick out, bringing the spine into a J-shape	✗ Tucking the tailbone
✓ Gradually increasing the intensity of and varying the exercises included in your workouts over time	✗ Doing the same workout at the same intensity over and over again
✓ Doing high-intensity interval training	✗ Logging long hours of cardio exercise each week
✓ Prioritizing stretching, strength training, and anaerobic exercise (such as intervals)	✗ Sticking to one category of exercise

TIME TAKEN, TIME SAVED

When you take one minute out of every fifteen to stand up or change positions while working at your desk, you'll improve your bone health, burn more calories, work more muscles, and burn more fat—all of which likely lessen your risk of dying prematurely.[4]

Healing Principle 5

Enjoy the Sun and Get Your Vitamin D

At a Glance

✓ Just as plants need sunlight to grow, you need sunlight to thrive.

✓ Regular, sensible sun exposure dramatically lowers your risk of cancer and heart disease and is the ideal way to get your vitamin D.

✓ In winter, use tanning beds without electromagnetic ballasts or take oral vitamin D_3.

✓ Testing your blood levels of vitamin D regularly is the best way to check whether you have an adequate amount.

F ew things feel better than sitting in a sunny spot, absorbing the warmth of the sun's rays. Unfortunately, due to decades of professional and media misinformation, you probably have been told the sun is harmful to your health.

As a result, you have likely been avoiding the midday sun and slathering yourself with high-SPF sunscreen when you do choose to be out in it. You may even be afraid of the sun's rays and go to great lengths to avoid them at all times. And who could blame you? The headlines about sun-related melanoma would make anyone want to hide under a rock.

Unfortunately, avoiding sunshine deprives you of the sun's truly staggering health-promoting properties. You probably already know that exposure to the sun prompts your skin to produce vitamin D. That's just one benefit. In a way, you are like a solar cell—you derive energy from the sun. Just as plants require sunlight to grow well, you require solar energy to thrive. A well-documented example is seasonal affective disorder (SAD)—the form of depression that occurs in winter, when people don't have access to regular bright sunlight. Science has yet to uncover the full range of the sun's benefits, but rest assured, more exist.

Here are six noteworthy ones, some of which you may never have heard of. Sunlight exposure can:

- Provide you with a healthful, cosmetically appealing tan
- Help reduce pain by improving your mood and releasing endorphins
- Help you burn fat more efficiently[1]
- Improve your evening alertness and help regulate your sleep cycles[2]
- Release nitric oxide,[3] a chemical transmitter stored in your skin, which is crucial for maintaining healthy blood pressure,[4] preventing atherosclerosis,[5] and modulating immune system function[6]

• Treat certain skin diseases such as psoriasis,[7] vitiligo,[8] atopic dermatitis,[9] and scleroderma[10]

All these benefits, from merely exposing your skin to the sun! Getting out in the sun truly is Effortless Healing. And that's just the beginning.

Benefits of Vitamin D

A mong all the health benefits of sensible sunlight exposure, vitamin D, which is produced by your skin in response to UVB radiation, is the most important. Vitamin D influences an estimated 10 percent of all the genes in your body. That makes it crucial for maintaining your health!

Vitamin D plays a major role in preventing cardiovascular disease, as by triggering your skin to release nitric oxide, it helps to significantly reduce hypertension and risk of heart attack and stroke.

Vitamin D also works in tandem with vitamin K (more on page 145) to help the body absorb calcium from food, then direct it away from arteries (where it can lead to hardening of the arteries, a dangerous precursor to heart disease) and toward the skeleton.

A 2008 study that followed nearly 1,800 men for approximately five years found that those with low levels of vitamin D (less than 15 ng/ml) were significantly more likely to develop cardiovascular disease than those with levels greater than 15 ng/ml; the risk was higher the lower the blood serum levels were.[11] As cardiovascular disease is still the number-one killer (just slightly ahead of cancer) in the United States,[12] this major benefit has the power to save a lot of lives.

Tragically, about 70 percent of Americans, and up to one

billion people worldwide, have unhealthy levels of vitamin D. Here are some of the side effects of having too-low vitamin D levels:

- Two recent studies of critically ill children found that vitamin D deficiency is very common in sick children and is associated with worse outcomes and extended hospital stays.[13] Earlier studies had already linked vitamin D deficiency to worse outcomes in critically ill adults.[14]

- Frail seniors with low levels of vitamin D have an increased risk of death, according to Oregon State University researchers.[15]

- More than two hundred epidemiological studies have tested and confirmed theories linking vitamin D deficiency to cancer. Breast cancer has even been described as a "vitamin D deficiency syndrome." Previous research showed that optimizing vitamin D levels can cut in half the risk for sixteen different types of cancer, including pancreatic, lung, ovarian, breast, prostate, and skin cancers.

- A number of studies show that vitamin D may even lower your risk of cavities.[16]

Perhaps vitamin D's biggest benefit is that it may lower your risk of dying from *any* cause. Truly, the health benefits of vitamin D are so astounding that I strongly believe optimizing its levels may be one of the most important things you can do to improve and maintain your health.

In my practice, I have used vitamin D supplementation and sensible sun exposure to treat patients with a wide array of conditions, including prostate cancer, depression, autism, rheumatoid arthritis, asthma, eczema, and digestive disorders.

One such patient was James, who had suffered with Crohn's disease for ten years. He had tried several diet modifications and prescription medications, but never seemed to get off the roller coaster of feeling slightly better, then having a major relapse a few months later. His Crohn's even landed him in the hospital on multiple occasions.

James, a computer programmer, spent most of his time indoors. He began prioritizing spending more time outdoors in full sun and taking 3,000 IU of vitamin D_3 per day. Within eight weeks, he was able to go off prednisone entirely. After six months of increased vitamin D_3 intake and sun exposure, his bowels were functioning normally, his skin lesions had healed, and his energy soared.

How can one vitamin have so many benefits?

Vitamin D influences DNA through vitamin D receptors (VDRs), which bind to specific locations of the human genome. Scientists have identified *nearly three thousand genes* that are influenced by vitamin D levels, and VDRs have been found throughout the human body. Is it any wonder that, no matter what disease or condition is investigated, vitamin D appears to play a crucial role?

A partial explanation lies in the fact that vitamin D is not actually a vitamin but a powerful steroid hormone precursor. Vitamin D_3 is not found in most foods but influences virtually every cell in your body. Raising your vitamin D levels is easily one of nature's most potent cancer prevention strategies.

But Won't Sun Exposure Open the Door to Melanoma?

A lot of bad press links sun exposure to skin cancer, but in fact, there is plenty of evidence to the contrary. Before we discuss melanoma, however, let's review the three most common types of skin cancer. Each one is named for the type of cells affected:

- **Basal cell carcinoma (BCC).** BCC begins in the basal cell layer of the skin, typically on the face. It is the most common form of skin cancer and the most common type of cancer in humans. It is also the least likely skin cancer to spread.[17]

- **Squamous cell carcinoma (SCC).** SCC begins in the squamous cells, typically on the face, neck, ears, lips, and backs of hands. It tends to grow and spread a bit more than BCC.

- **Melanoma.** Melanoma begins in the melanocytes, the cells that produce the pigment melanin (responsible for your tan). Melanin protects the deeper layers of skin from excess radiation. Melanoma is more likely than other types of skin cancer to spread to other parts of the body, and it causes more deaths than any other type of skin cancer. Your risk of dying from it, however, pales in comparison to your risk of dying from cardiovascular disease.

Robert Heaney, M.D., a professor of endocrinology at Creighton University, is one of the leading vitamin D experts in the world. There is almost no evidence to support the idea that sun exposure increases your risk of melanoma, he says, and in fact there is compelling evidence to support the opposite:[18]

- An epidemic of melanoma has broken out among *indoor* workers. These workers get three to nine times *less* solar UV exposure than outdoor workers get, yet only indoor workers have increasing rates of melanoma—and the rates have been increasing since before 1940.[19]

- Melanoma is more common in regions of the body that are not exposed to the sun than in those that are. In 75 percent of cases it occurs on relatively unexposed sites.

- Melanoma is frequently misdiagnosed—the "rising rates of

melanoma" that you may have heard about are actually rising rates of minimal, noncancerous lesions.[20]

- Melanoma mortality actually decreases with greater sun exposure.[21]
- Melanoma incidence has been increasing, but at the same time people have been listening to the experts and decreasing their sun exposure. The rise in incidence is most likely related to decreased vitamin D levels, as there is good evidence that vitamin D retards the risk of melanoma.

But if sun exposure doesn't cause melanoma, then what does?

The *Real* Role of the Sun in Melanoma

In all serious diseases, multiple interacting factors—such as poor nutrition, environmental toxins, stress, and inadequate sleep—cause the immune system to go awry.

A frequently overlooked nutrition factor, though, is the ratio of omega-6 to omega-3 fats. In 2001 a comprehensive review published by the National Academy of Sciences showed that optimizing the omega-6:omega-3 ratio is instrumental in reducing the occurrence of skin cancers.[22] And an Australian study published over twenty years ago found that those who regularly ate fish, naturally high in omega-3 fats, showed a 40 percent reduction of melanoma. Your ancient ancestors consumed these fats in a ratio ranging from 5:1 to 1:1. With all the industrial food processing today, however, that ratio has blossomed to 20:1 to 50:1.

So it's important not only to consume more omega-3 fats but also to dramatically reduce consumption of omega-6 fats. Doing so will powerfully reduce your risk for acquiring melanoma. In addition, eating more nutrient-dense foods, like sunflower sprouts and fermented vegetables (as I suggest in Healing Principle 2), will provide your body with beneficial micronutrients that offer powerful antioxidant protection against too much omega-6.

As mentioned by Dr. Heaney, the sun does appear to play a significant role, but not the role you have heard about: melanoma may actually signify that you are getting too little of it! Studies show that melanoma mortality actually *decreases* after UV exposure. Additionally, melanoma lesions do not predominate on sun-exposed skin, which is why sunscreens have proven ineffective in preventing it. Exposure to sunlight, particularly UVB—or rather, the vitamin D that the body produces in response to UVB radiation—is protective against melanoma.

The bottom line: if you avoid the sun, your risk for vitamin D deficiency skyrockets. That will increase your odds of developing melanoma, as well as the two main causes of death, heart disease and cancer. The risks associated with insufficient vitamin D are *far greater* than those posed by basal cell or squamous cell carcinomas, which are fairly benign by comparison.

Sun Exposure

One key to getting vitamin D from the sun is to imagine your skin as solar panels. If you put a shirt over a solar panel, it will not generate any electricity.

Many people are under the mistaken idea that they can get enough vitamin D from exposing their forearms and face for a few minutes a day. But exposing our faces and forearms is grossly inadequate to moving vitamin D levels into a healthy range. For optimal benefit, strive to have at least 40 percent of your skin uncovered.

Most people living in the United States are able to get enough UVB from the sun only about six months out of the year. The rest of the time the UVB that penetrates the atmosphere isn't sufficient to produce vitamin D—even if you stay outside all day long with virtually no clothes on (impossible in a Chicago winter!). (Please see www.mercola.com/article/vitamin-d-resources.htm for a helpful graphic on vitamin D synthesis.)

The other challenge is that most people have to work, and typically our jobs keep us indoors five days a week. You can get sun exposure during the workday by walking to work and by taking lunch breaks outside—but keep in mind that the more skin you expose, the more vitamin D you will produce. A 2014 Australian study found that skin exposure was the most important factor in vitamin D levels, even greater than latitude and season.[23]

The production of D_3 in skin varies depending on many different factors:

Age

Typically, the older you get after 50, the less able your body is to convert UVB radiation to vitamin D.

Reflection

Nearby water, snow, ice, or glass may amplify the number of UVB rays hitting your skin.

Altitude

The higher the altitude, the greater the intensity of sunlight, and the less time you'll need to produce vitamin D.

Season

When the sun is lower than 50 degrees above the horizon, nearly all UVB rays are deflected by the atmosphere.

Skin Color and/or Current Tan Level

The darker your skin, the more sun exposure you will need to maintain optimal vitamin D levels.

Cloud Cover and Smog

Both block UVB rays.

Sunscreen

Nearly all sunscreens prevent UVB rays from penetrating skin.

Latitude

Your location on the Earth affects the height of the sun in the sky and thus how many UVB rays reach the ground.

Time of Day

The higher the sun is in the sky, the more UVB rays will reach the ground. The ideal times for producing vitamin D through sun exposure are when the sun is highest. If it's too low, the ozone will filter out most UVB rays.

Ozone Layer

Ozone filters UVBs. You can produce your daily dose of vitamin D in just a few minutes where ozone is thin— then cover up quickly so you don't get burned.

Weight

The heavier you are, the more vitamin D you require.

Guidelines for Sensible Sun Exposure

If you have light-colored skin, the color of your skin will tell you when you've had enough sun and it's time to get in the shade (or to cover up using a long-sleeved shirt, pants, and a hat). Stay out just long enough that your skin turns the very lightest shade of pink or one shade darker if you are dark skinned. Continuing UV exposure beyond the minimal dose required to produce skin redness will not increase your vitamin D production any further. But it will increase your risk of skin damage, photoaging, and benign skin cancers. (And, again, if you are still concerned about melanoma, remember that sun exposure is actually associated with a lower incidence of melanoma, and that many melanomas occur in skin that has not been exposed to the sun.)

In Caucasian skin, this will typically occur within ten to twenty minutes of ultraviolet exposure during ideal conditions. It can take three to six times longer for darkly pigmented skin to reach the proper concentration of skin vitamin D. Why is skin color a factor? Because melanin, the pigment that gives skin its color, is a potent filter of ultraviolet radiation, including the vitamin-D-producing UVB rays. So if you or your immediate ancestors are from Africa, India, or the Middle East, and you have dark skin, know that you require longer bouts of sunbathing without sunscreen to maintain adequate levels of vitamin D.

The first few days of the season, when it is warm enough to start wearing shorts and T-shirts, you should actually limit your exposure to the sun. This will allow your body's pigment cells to rev up the ability to produce the protective pigmentation that not only gives you a tan but helps protect you against overexposure to the sun.

If you tend to burn, you will want to limit your initial exposure to a few minutes, especially if it is in the middle of summer. The more tanned your skin gets, and/or the more tanned you want to become, the longer you can stay in the sun. If it is early or late in the season and/or you are a dark-skinned individual, you could likely safely stay thirty minutes on your initial exposure. Always err on the side of caution, however, and let it be your primary goal to never get sunburned.

Protect Your Face and Eyes

The skin on your face is typically much thinner than it is on other areas on your body. It is also a relatively small surface area, so it will not contribute much to vitamin D production. I strongly recommend that you protect this fragile area; facial skin is at a much higher risk for cosmetic photo damage and premature wrinkling. Use a safe sunblock on this area, or wear a cap that always keeps your eyes in the shade, as I do when I'm outside seeking to increase my vitamin D levels. Sometimes we forget about the simplest things, like wearing a hat.

Sunscreens and Moisturizers

Use no sunscreens when soaking in the rays for this purpose. If you need to moisturize your skin, use a safe, *non*-SPF cream. Organic coconut oil will also moisturize your skin, and at the same time benefit you metabolically by reducing your appetite and improving your thyroid function. Remember, if the moisturizer you use has an SPF value, it will block UVB rays and will not allow your body to produce vitamin D. If you stay outdoors for the rest of the day, stay in the shade and appropriately cover exposed skin with clothing. If you still want to be in the open sun, use a nontoxic lotion with SPF15 for uncovered skin. Just be sure to stay on the safe side of burning!

If you do use a sunscreen, please choose the product carefully. Many sunscreens contain chemicals you don't want absorbed into your body. According to the Environmental Working Group's 2014 Sunscreen Guide, about 75 percent of sunscreens contain potentially harmful ingredients, such as oxybenzone and retinyl palmitate.[24]

When selecting a sunscreen, look for one that includes zinc oxide and/or titanium dioxide: these two naturally occurring minerals will protect your skin from ultraviolet rays by forming

PROTECT YOUR SKIN FROM THE INSIDE OUT

Using an "internal sunscreen" is an alternative to topical sunblock agents.

Dr. John Cannell of the Vitamin D Council claims that taking 10,000 IU per day for several months before you start sunbathing will help prevent sunburn. Most people who have high levels of 25(OH)D—the precursor of vitamin D known as 25-hydroxyvitamin D, which your kidneys convert into a usable form of vitamin D and that vitamin D blood tests seek to measure—will tell you that their skin reacts differently to excess sun.

In addition, astaxanthin—a potent antioxidant derived from algae—has been found to offer effective protection against sun damage when taken as a daily supplement. It can also be used topically, and a number of sunscreen products contain it. Some sunscreens are also starting to use astaxanthin as an ingredient to help protect skin from potential sun damage.

a physical barrier and reflecting and scattering UV rays away from your body. Other ingredients that are beneficial in a sunscreen are natural moisturizers (such as jojoba oil, coconut oil, or shea butter) and antioxidants (such as green tea extract or astaxanthin). I am proud of the all-natural sunscreen we sell on Mercola.com. For other options, and for the most recent version of its sunscreen guide, visit the Environmental Working Group's site (www.ewg.org).

If You Get Sunburned

If you develop a sunburn, aloe vera is one of the best remedies. It is loaded with powerful glyconutrients that accelerate healing. It is best to use the gel fresh from a leaf off a plant, but commercial products are available that have active aloe in them. Look for one that bears the seal of the International Aloe Science Council

(IASC), which certifies products that contain true, unadulterated aloe vera. Ideally, you won't need it because you are using these safe tanning guidelines, but accidents do happen.

Avoid Tanning Through a Window

Being exposed to bright sunshine while indoors is certainly good for your emotional health, but tanning through a window will not increase your vitamin D levels. The UVA rays have a long wavelength that easily penetrates materials, such as the earth's atmosphere and window glass. But the UVB wavelengths that produce vitamin D are much shorter and less energetic than UVA, and most are unable to penetrate window glass. When you're exposed to sunlight through windows—in your office, your home, or your car—you get UVA but virtually none of the beneficial UVB.

Many people are surprised to learn that tanning through a window will actually increase their risk for certain skin cancers. Not only do UVA rays destroy vitamin D_3, they also increase oxidative stress. UVA exposure is one of the primary culprits behind skin cancer, and it increases photoaging of your skin. It's also what causes you to tan. Most people don't realize you can actually get vitamin D without significantly darkening your skin, because the UVB wavelength does not stimulate the melanin pigment to produce a tan.

Normally, when you get tanned from outdoor sun exposure, you're getting both UVA and UVB at the same time, as sunlight is approximately 95 percent UVA and 5 percent UVB. This ratio provides a natural balance, as the UVB rays produce vitamin D, which then helps protect the body from the UVA rays, which penetrate the skin more deeply, are responsible for photoaging, and trigger damage that can lead to skin cancer. But when you are indoors and expose yourself to sunlight filtered through window glass, you are increasing your risk for skin cancer, because while the UVAs are effectively destroying your vitamin D_3 levels, you're getting none of the benefits of UVB. This is one reason why many people who drive long hours in their cars develop skin cancer on the arm next to the car window.

Tanning Beds

Sensible sun exposure is undoubtedly the best way to get vitamin D. There is little doubt in my mind that getting vitamin D naturally from the sun is far superior than swallowing a vitamin D pill. But it's impractical for most people for major portions of the year. By using a tanning bed, you can simulate the same process that occurs when you get vitamin D from the sun.

Most tanning equipment uses magnetic ballasts, but they are well-known sources of electromagnetic fields, which can contribute to cancer. If you hear a loud buzzing noise while you are in a tanning bed, you know it has a magnetic ballast system. I strongly recommend you avoid this type of bed and choose instead a tanning bed that uses an electronic ballast. These machines are nearly silent.

The other factor to consider when selecting a tanning bed is the type of light it emits. There are two main categories of ultraviolet radiation—UVA and UVB. Each has a different wavelength and affects your body in different ways. UVB is the form that stimulates your skin to produce vitamin D_3. When UVB radiation strikes the skin surface, the skin converts a cholesterol derivative into vitamin D_3. Most people don't realize you can actually get vitamin D without significantly darkening the skin, because the UVB wavelength does not stimulate the melanin pigment to produce a tan.

UVA radiation works differently. It's what causes you to tan. It penetrates the skin more deeply and triggers a tan. But it does not produce vitamin D_3. In fact, it destroys some of the vitamin D that is formed on the skin by UVB.

So you'll want to find a tanning bed that emits a good percentage of UVB rays. Beds tend to emit between 3 and 10 percent UVB—the higher the better. Some beds emit UVB only.

These beds aren't very popular, as UVB rays don't provide a tan. Most in the tanning industry value UVA rays above all others as they are the ones that lead to a tan. So you will likely have to do some searching to find one (and make sure it uses an electronic ballast). The best way to find out if your local salon has what you need is to call and ask to speak to the manager.

Once you are positioned in the tanning bed, protect your face. Your facial skin is thinner than the skin on the rest of your body, so it is more susceptible to sun damage. Stay in the bed just long enough for your skin to turn slightly pink, which is the visible cue that your skin has started to produce vitamin D. Just as with natural sunbathing, you don't want to stay long enough to get a burn.

You can purchase a tanning bed, but they typically cost over $1,000 and won't be an option for everyone.

Vitamin D Supplements

As I've said, the best way to increase your vitamin D level is by sensible sun exposure, and a UVB tanning bed comes in second. But if those are not options for you, then you're well advised to take an oral supplement.

The most common question would be, how much should you take? The best answer is, whatever dose causes your 25-hydroxyvitamin D blood test to be between 50 and 70 ng/ml. This is true for anyone, from newborns to centenarians.

Individual responses to vitamin D vary dramatically, so the

best way to know if your dose is correct is to do a blood test. A safe starting dose for most adults is 5,000 IU a day. In the past there was much concern over vitamin D toxicity, but we now know that it was misplaced: there is virtually no danger of toxicity at this safe level. In fact, a surprising number of people need more than 20,000 IU of vitamin D daily to reach ideal blood levels.

The only way to know for sure if you are supplementing with the right amount is to have your blood levels tested. I rarely recommend you rush out to the doctor's office, but you require a blood test to accurately determine your Vitamin D levels. I covered this in detail in Chapter 2—refer back to page 26 for more detailed instructions.

You also need to make sure you're taking the right kind of vitamin D. Most people don't know that D_2—the synthetic version commonly prescribed by doctors—is not as potent as D_3. Each microgram of oral vitamin D_3 is about five times more effective in raising serum D than an equivalent amount of vitamin D_2.

If You Take Vitamin D Supplements, Take Vitamin K₂, Too

If you're taking oral vitamin D supplements, it is wise to take vitamin K_2 as well. Vitamin K_2 helps move calcium into the proper areas in your body. It helps shift calcium from blood vessels and soft tissues, where it could otherwise harden them to bones and teeth to increase their density.

Vitamin K_2 deficiency is actually what produces the symptoms of vitamin D toxicity, which include inappropriate calcification that can lead to hardening of the arteries.[25] When you take vitamin D, your body creates more vitamin K_2-dependent proteins that move calcium around in your body. Without vitamin K_2, those proteins remain inactivated, so the benefits of those proteins remain unrealized. So remember, if you take supplemental vitamin D, you're creating an increased demand for K_2. Together, these two nutrients help strengthen your bones and improve your heart health.

While the ideal or optimal ratios between vitamin D and vitamin K_2 have yet to be pinpointed, Dr. Kate Rhéaume-Bleue, author of *Vitamin K_2 and the Calcium Paradox: How a Little-Known Vitamin Could Save Your Life,* suggests you may benefit from 100 to 250 micrograms (mcg) of K_2 daily.

Visit GrassrootsHealth.net for a chart that suggests how much vitamin D_3 to take in order to achieve optimal levels, based on your starting level.

Your Effortless Action Plan

1. *Whenever the weather is warm enough, expose at least 40 percent of your body to the sun's rays, using safe-tanning guidelines, for long enough to turn your skin pink (if you're light-skinned) or a shade darker (if you're dark-skinned).*

2. *Investigate safe tanning options in your area for times of year when the sun isn't strong enough to produce vitamin D.*

3. *If you aren't able to get adequate amounts of sun exposure or spend time in a tanning bed, consider taking 5,000 IU of vitamin D_3 and 100 to 250 mcg of K_2 daily.*

4. *Monitor your levels of vitamin D by getting your blood tested at least twice a year, and adjust your sun exposure and supplement levels to get your blood levels to between 50 and 70 ng/ml.*

HEALERS	HURTERS
✓ Exposing at least 40 percent of your skin to the sun just until it turns pink (or one shade darker, if you're dark-skinned)	✗ Wearing sunscreen all the time or clothes covering most of your skin
✓ Sunbathing at close to solar noon (1:00 p.m. during daylight saving time), as UVB rays are most prevalent then	✗ Getting sun exposure through glass or sunbathing when the sun is low in the sky (and UVB rays are least abundant)
✓ Taking oral vitamin D_3 supplements	✗ Taking vitamin D_2 supplements
✓ Adding vitamin K_2 if taking oral vitamin D_3	✗ Taking vitamin D_3 supplements without also taking vitamin K_2
✓ Using mineral-based sunscreens when you must be in direct sunlight with little clothes coverage	✗ Using chemical-based sunscreen
✓ Getting your 25(OH)D levels tested—with the help of a doctor—regularly till in good range then at least annually after that	✗ Not knowing your blood levels of vitamin D

Healing Principle 6

Let Your Gut Flourish

At a Glance

✓ The bacteria in your gut outnumber the human cells in your body ten to one.

✓ These bacteria offer crucial aid in digestion, germ protection, and mood regulation.

✓ Many aspects of modern living can be harmful to the beneficial bacteria in your gut.

✓ Your body and brain function will suffer if your beneficial bacteria are not optimal.

✓ Eating fermented foods is a delicious way to nurture your friendly bacteria.

✓ When the probiotic population in your gut is thriving, these tiny microbes perform multiple functions that help keep you healthy and happy—really!

Your body is literally teeming with bacteria. And this is an extremely good thing! These tiny organisms that make up your gut flora, or the microbiome, exert a truly profound influence on your health. Their importance cannot be overstated.

Ninety percent of the genetic material in your body is not yours. It's from the bacteria that are primarily living in your gut. You have about 100 trillion bacteria living in your gut and only 10 trillion cells, so collectively they outnumber you ten to one. These bacteria provide a large number of incredibly important benefits such as:

- Optimizing your immune system and helping you resist infections
- Helping you digest food and absorb nutrients
- Detoxifying heavy metals and chemicals you have been exposed to
- Providing B vitamins and vitamin K_2
- Balancing your nervous system by serving as a source of neurotransmitters

These beneficial bacteria also train your immune system to distinguish between pathogens (disease-causing microbes) and nonharmful microbes. They prevent your immune system from overreacting, which is the genesis of allergies. Furthermore, your intestinal health can have a profound influence on your mental health. Your gut is quite literally your second brain, as it originates from the same type of tissue as your brain!

The gastrointestinal tract is now considered one of the most complex microbial ecosystems on earth. You may have a basic awareness that the microbes in your gut affect your digestion. But their influence extends far beyond that to your brain, heart, skin, mood, weight . . . and the list goes on and on.

In many ways, your health is foundationally rooted in your

gut bacteria, both in terms of maintaining emotional and physical wellness, and in terms of preventing chronic disease. When gut microbes are abundant, they work tirelessly on processes that support your body's natural ability to heal itself. Letting them do much of the heavy lifting for you is truly effortless. (Now if only we could train them to answer e-mails and scrub toilets!)

Beneficial bacteria are so crucial to health that researchers have compared them to "a newly recognized organ" and have even suggested we consider ourselves a type of "meta-organism," with multiple environments within our body—such as our mouth, our gut, and our skin—each of which hosts its own unique population of microbiota.

Your Gut: More Than Just a Food Processing Factory

If you think about your gut at all, you might think of it as a simple mechanism whose job is to digest food, but this is actually just one small role it plays. Rather than merely responding to input (like food), your gut actually initiates a staggering number of actions in your body. In a very real sense, you have *two brains*, one inside your skull and one in your gut. So nourishing your gut flora is extremely important, from cradle to grave.

A Second Brain

You actually have two nervous systems:

- Central nervous system, composed of your brain and spinal cord
- Enteric nervous system, the intrinsic nervous system of your gastrointestinal tract

Interestingly, these two organs are created out of the same type of tissue. During fetal development, one part turns into your central nervous system while the other develops into your enteric nervous system. These two systems are connected via the vagus nerve, the tenth cranial nerve that runs from your brain stem down to your abdomen.

You might believe that your brain directs how your body functions, but your gut actually sends far more information to your brain than your brain sends to your gut. The vagus nerve is the mechanism your gut flora use to send messages to your brain.

Yes, your brain sends instructions to your gut, but it's a two-way street. Your gut also sends instructions to your brain. And while science hasn't determined exactly how the communication is initiated, research suggests that the microbes in your gut play an important role.

For example, a 2013 study by researchers at UCLA found that women who consumed yogurt twice a day had significantly different brain function and connections between regions of the brain than women who either ate a version of yogurt that contained no probiotics or who ate no yogurt at all.[1] The findings suggest that the number and type of probiotics you have in your gut affect the way your brain works and is organized. (For my thoughts on the best type of yogurt, see Healing Principle 9.)

At this point, most other studies of the link between microbiome and brain function have been conducted on animals, but the results are fascinating. Specific strains of probiotics have been found to reduce stress hormones and behaviors associated with anxiety and depression,[2] and to reduce symptoms of anxiety in mice with colitis.[3]

To put it in more concrete terms: you've probably experienced the visceral sensation of butterflies in your stomach when you're nervous, or you've had an upset stomach when you were angry or stressed. But the flip side is also true: problems in your gut can directly impact your mental health, paving the way for anxiety and depression.

While we don't yet know exactly how this link between gut health and mental health functions, researchers at Texas Tech University have found that different strains of probiotics produce different neurochemicals, such as GABA (which reduces stress and anxiety), serotonin (which reduces aggressive behavior and promotes sleep), and dopamine (which plays a role in focus, pleasure, and motivation).[4] It is likely that these chemicals, traveling between your gut and your brain via your vagus nerve, influence mental health.

> Optimizing your gut flora is far superior to getting a flu shot.

The Immune System

In addition to acting as a second brain, your gut also houses 80 percent of your immune system. (Your skin and your lymph nodes are the other major players in immunity.) It is your body's primary tool for fighting infections.

As I briefly mentioned earlier, your gut flora work to keep your immune system strong in a few ways:

- They keep potentially harmful invaders at bay primarily by taking up space in your digestive tract, protecting against overgrowth of microorganisms that could cause disease.
- Your microbiome also "teaches" your immune system which items to attack and which to tolerate. They help neutralize pathogenic (disease-causing) bacteria that you may be exposed to through food.

- They help manage allergies. Infants who have a less diverse population of microbiotics have an increased risk of developing allergies when they grow older.[5]
- They fuel another piece of your immune system, the thymus gland, which provides cell-mediated immunity through the release of T cells.
- They are also excellent detoxifiers, helping your body process and expel toxins that could otherwise build up and compromise your health.

Digestion

Even with all these immune and other benefits, your gut flora's power to aid in digestion shouldn't be overlooked. If your internal environment isn't well stocked with the beneficial bacteria needed to break down your food properly, your body won't be able to assimilate all those important nutrients you're consuming.

Gut Bacteria That Need Help

How can you tell whether your health is suffering from a lack of healthy gut bacteria? The following symptoms are all possible signs that unhealthy bacteria have taken over too much real estate in your gut. The more symptoms you have, the more likely that you have a less-than-ideal gut flora population.

- Gas and bloating
- Constipation or diarrhea
- Fatigue
- Nausea
- Headaches
- Sugar cravings, and cravings for refined carbs

- Depression or low mood
- Frequent infections
- Insomnia

Please take these warning signs seriously, since a healthy gut is one of your best defenses against disease. Imbalances in gut flora are actually quite common, considering how vulnerable gut bacteria are to environmental insults.

Lifestyle Stresses on the Gut

Lifestyle can and does influence your inner environment on a daily basis. Your gut bacteria are extremely sensitive to:

Antibiotics Yes, antibiotics do kill bacteria that can make you ill. But they can also imbalance the population of friendly bacteria in your gut, leaving you more vulnerable to subsequent illness. Eighty percent of the antibiotics distributed in the United States are fed to farm animals, so if the meat you're eating isn't organic, you can safely assume you are getting a dose of antibiotics with each bite, and are also potentially being exposed to antibiotic-resistant bacteria.

Chlorinated water If you are drinking unfiltered, chlorinated tap water, remember that chlorine kills not only water-borne pathogens but also your beneficial bacteria.

Antibacterial soap A large population of friendly bacteria lives on your skin, which is one of the main reasons skin-to-skin contact is recommended for newborns and premature babies. (It doesn't just feel good—hugging this way also transmits these tiny helpers to your offspring.) These bacteria ward off invaders that may find their way into your system through cuts in your skin. Antibacterial soap targets these friendly microbes, too. In addition, most antibacterial soaps contain triclosan, which may alter your hormones[6] or interfere with your muscles. Triclosan has been linked to heart disease and heart failure.[7] Even the FDA has become wary of triclosan—at the end of 2013, it proposed a rule that would require manufacturers of products that contain it to prove that those products provide more benefit than simply washing with soap and water.[8]

When you are bathing, I recommend that you use plain soap, as little as possible, as all soap removes most of the natural oil in the sebum of your skin. Sebum, produced by your sebaceous glands, not only helps prevent your hair and skin from drying out but also provides an important barrier of protection against infections.

Agricultural chemicals Herbicides designed to kill weeds are heralded by their manufacturers to be innocuous to humans. But they are *not* innocuous to your microflora. When you eat foods contaminated with herbicides—in particular, glyphosate, the active ingredient in the ubiquitous pesticide Roundup—they can enter your cells and target your beneficial bacteria.

Pollution Contaminants in the air have recently been linked to gastrointestinal disorders. One study revealed that short-term exposure to air pollution may trigger abdominal pain in young adults as well as even more serious diseases, like inflammatory bowel disease.[9]

The Most Important Factor in Healthy Gut Flora: Diet

P oor diet—particularly one that is loaded with processed foods and sugar—is the number-one enemy of healthy gut bacteria. Cleaning up your diet is essential to good health—I give plenty more details about how to do it in Healing Principles 2 and 9. But with regard to your microbiome, here are the tolls associated with the processed foods that so many consume.

- **Sugar.** Processed foods are typically loaded with sugar. Sugar compromises your beneficial gut bacteria by providing the preferred fuel for pathogenic bacteria. It also contributes to chronic inflammation throughout your body, including your brain.
- **Refined grains.** Processed foods are also often loaded with refined grains, which your body rapidly converts into sugar.
- **Genetically engineered (GE) ingredients.** The majority of processed foods contain GE ingredients (primarily corn, soy, and canola), which are particularly detrimental to beneficial bacteria. Eating genetically engineered corn may turn your gut flora into a sort of "living pesticide factory," essentially manufacturing Bt-toxin *from within* your digestive system on a continuing basis.[10] Moreover, beneficial gut bacteria are very sensitive to residual glyphosate, the active ingredient in Roundup.[11] Glyphosate alters and destroys beneficial gut flora in animals, as evidenced by the increasing instances of lethal botulism in cattle.[12]

Eating a *healthy diet* helps the beneficial gut bacteria flourish, which results in the real "magic" of restoring your health. And once you teach yourself how to eat this way, the incredible vitality you will likely feel will make choosing healthy foods truly effortless.

One of my readers, Arno, was sixty-nine and eating a typical diet heavy in processed foods and grains, when he took a course of antibiotics after having an infected tooth extracted. The antibiotics wiped out his already imperiled beneficial bacteria population, and he developed extreme diarrhea—hourly episodes with blood in the stool. The MDs he consulted (four in total) said his condition was life-threatening, and all suggested that he take another round of antibiotics. Instead, Arno chose to flood his system with probiotics. He consumed fermented foods, such as natto, kefir, yogurt, tempeh, and sauerkraut, every day. In three days, his diarrhea was gone. Since then, he has continued to eat probiotic foods daily and has improved the quality of his food with many more raw vegetables and leafy greens. He is happy to report that not only has his digestion been greatly enhanced, but he hasn't had a cold in the five years since.

The Benefits of Restoring Your Gut Flora Balance

Tending to your microflora—consistently reseeding your gut with healthy bacteria—pays dividends in multiple areas of health, many of which might surprise you. It may be crucial to the prevention of virtually all disease, from coughs, colds, and flus; to autoimmune disorders; to psychiatric disturbances; and even to cancer. If you have any of the following conditions, you need to promote the growth of beneficial bacteria in your gut.

Behavior Issues

Recent animal research has found a link between gut bacteria and behavior. Mice with a poorly populated bacterial population were found to be more likely to engage in "high-risk behavior" than mice with healthy gut flora. This altered behavior was accompanied by neurochemical changes in the animals' brains. Researchers believe that the expression of certain genes that affect behavior is connected to bacteria in the gut.

BACTERIA AND AUTISM:
A MISSING LINK?

Most of the microbes that comprise an infant's gut flora are acquired during birth. However, babies born via C-section don't acquire their mother's vaginal and intestinal microbes at birth. Their gut flora is established primarily through contact with their parents' skin and is much less robust than that of babies born vaginally. This explains why babies born by C-section have higher rates of asthma, allergy, and autoimmune disorders.[13]

If you are currently pregnant or become pregnant, it's even more important for you to prioritize tending to your microbiome, as it may be one of the most important steps you can take for your child.

The rate of autism has risen dramatically since I graduated medical school, from 1 in 10,000 to now less than 1 in 50. There is compelling evidence that the rapid rise in autism is at least partially related to gut flora. If an infant's gut flora is less than optimal, instead of being a source of nourishment, it becomes a major source of toxicity. Pathogenic organisms, left unchecked by the absence of friendly microbes, damage the integrity of the gut wall. This allows all sorts of toxins and microbes to flow into the bloodstream of the infant and penetrate its brain, which appears to lead to autism or autismlike symptoms.

Researchers—particularly Dr. Natasha Campbell-McBride, a neurologist, the mother of an autistic child, and the author of *Gut and Psychology Syndrome*—are seeing an increased risk of children with abnormal gut flora developing such disorders as ADHD, learning disabilities, and autism, particularly if they are vaccinated *before* restoring balance to their gut flora. To get a solid understanding of just how this connection works, I highly recommend that you read Dr. Campbell-McBride's book. In my opinion, it is essential reading for all parents and parents-to-be.

Immunity

Establishment of normal gut flora in the first twenty days or so of life plays a crucial role in appropriate maturation of a baby's immune system. Babies who develop abnormal gut flora, by contrast, are left with compromised immune systems.

Obesity

The makeup of gut bacteria tends to differ in lean and obese people. In people who are obese or gain weight easily, studies show, gut flora is significantly less diverse than in those of normal weight.

Research also suggests that people are more likely to gain weight when their gut bacteria break down food inefficiently, enabling their bodies to absorb more calories. One reason fermented foods are so beneficial to weight loss is that they contain lactic acid bacteria—beneficial gut bacteria that can help you stay slim. This may be one reason breast-fed babies have a lower risk of obesity, as bifidobacteria flourish in the guts of breast-fed babies.

Obese people who drank a probiotic-rich fermented milk beverage for 12 weeks were able to reduce their abdominal fat by nearly 5 percent, and their subcutaneous fat by over 3 percent. In that study, the control group experienced no significant fat reductions at all—which earns one more gold star for probiotics. When pregnant women take probiotics from the first trimester through breastfeeding, they appear to lose weight more easily after childbirth.

Much more research shows that lean people tend to have higher amounts of various healthy bacteria than do obese people. The bottom line: if you are seeking to lose weight, restoring balance to your gut flora is a crucial piece of the puzzle.

Multiple Sclerosis

Multiple sclerosis is a chronic, degenerative disease of the nerves in the brain and spinal column, caused through an immune-mediated demyelination process. Myelin is the insulating, waxy substance around the nerves in the central nervous system; when the myelin is damaged by an autoimmune disease or similarly destructive process in the body, the function of those nerves deteriorates over time.

It may seem strange that microbes in the digestive tract could influence a disease of the brain and spinal column, but current research clearly shows that gut bacteria *do* play a vital role in triggering autoimmune demyelination; they also influence the immune system's inflammatory response.[14] And although the research is still new and ongoing into the possibility, there have been some indications that dietary changes could reverse MS in some individuals.[15]

Depression, Anxiety, and PTSD

Many experts describe the gut as the "second brain," as it produces more neurotransmitters than the actual brain. So improving beneficial bacteria in the gut may be the answer we've been looking for to address rampant mental health problems such as depression.

Remember, you have neurons both in your brain *and* in your gut—including neurons that produce neurotransmitters like serotonin. In fact, the greatest concentration of serotonin—which is involved in mood control, depression, and aggression—is found in your *intestines,* not in your brain!

This may well be one reason antidepressants, which raise serotonin levels in your *brain,* are often ineffective in treating depression, whereas proper dietary changes often do help.

In fact, a new arm of psychological science called psychobiotics promotes the medicinal use of probiotics that are known to affect neurotransmitters such as serotonin and dopamine. Even severe and chronic mental health problems, like post-traumatic stress disorder (PTSD), might be eliminated through the use of certain beneficial bacteria.[16]

One reason may be that many psychiatric illnesses have an association with low-level chronic inflammation.[17] And beneficial flora, studies have found, can modulate inflammation and restore healthy immunological function.[18] So by enhancing gut flora, we can lower the inflammation that is a factor in many psychiatric challenges.

Skin Issues

Signals from your gut flora are sent throughout your body and interact with organisms in your skin and gut. Researchers are now looking into how these interactions can help with skin conditions like dryness, improve collagen, and stabilize skin microflora to help with irritations.

At first it may seem strange that bacteria in your gut would play a role in skin health, but when you consider that your skin is literally bathed in bacteria, it's not such a stretch after all. Even after you wash, there are still one million bacteria living on every square centimeter of your skin. They are involved in a symbiotic relationship with you. The bacteria in the crook of your inner elbow, for instance, process the raw fats produced by your skin and in turn help moisturize the area.[19]

Beneficial bacteria play an important role in skin health. Beneficial bacteria supplementation, we know, can help treat and prevent eczema. Eczema, also known as atopic dermatitis, is more than just a skin problem; it signals a problem with the immune system. In fact, eczema is said to be one of the first signs of allergy during the first days of life. A recent study has found that children under two with eczema have triple the risk of developing asthma or hay fever as they get older than children who don't have eczema.[20]

If an infant or child struggles with eczema, providing them with beneficial bacteria is a great idea. If the child isn't eating solid foods yet, apply a probiotic powder to a parent's clean pinkie or a mother's nipple. Feed an older child probiotic foods such as yogurt, kefir, or sauerkraut. Probiotics can also be helpful for any infant born via C-section, as it would help the immune system to develop and mature.

Other useful ways to address eczema are to expose the eczema to sunlight; eliminate gluten and processed sugars from the person's diet; and make sure the consumption of omega-3 fats is optimal.

Cancer

Several types of cancer are linked to particular microbes. For example, the human papilloma virus (HPV) is a contributing factor in cervical cancer. But overall, the relationship between gut flora and cancer is far more complex.

Although we don't yet fully understand the mechanism, scientists are proving the link exists. A 2013 study by researchers at New York University School of Medicine, for example, found that patients with colorectal cancer had a less diverse population of gut bacteria than healthy people.[21] The simplest explanation may be that an imbalance in the bacterial population of the gut—too many bad bacteria, not enough of the friendly strains—creates the conditions for the disease to form and thrive.[22]

How to Nourish Your Gut with Food

How to Get Your Gut Flora Back in Balance

Consistently reseeding your gut with healthy bacteria may be crucial for help in the prevention of virtually all disease, as well as from coughs, colds, and flus; autoimmune disorders; psychiatric disturbances; and even cancer. The good news is that improving the health of your digestive system is a simple, straightforward process of achieving the right balance of good and bad gut bacteria. It's a matter of moving the right bacteria, in the right amounts, into permanent residence in your digestive tract. And doing that is very nearly effortless: you avoid sugars, chlorinated water, and processed foods, and you eat more fermented foods. In addition to being delicious, fermented foods have the added benefit of being powerful healers that you can create on your own with minimal investment and energy.

Simply eating more fermented foods is the best way to optimize your digestive health. Be sure to eat the traditionally made, unpasteurized versions. Healthy choices include fermented shredded vegetables and fermented unpasteurized dairy like yogurt and kefir. (See the Healers/Hurters box on page 173 for a full list.) Ideally you would make your yogurt or kefir yourself (kefir in particular is easy, I promise—see recipe on page 168), as most commercial versions are loaded with sugars and artificial flavors and sweeteners and are low in beneficial bacteria.

In most traditional cuisines, people eat some form of fermented food every day, as this was how they preserved food before refrigeration was available. For best results, you'll want to eat a bit of fermented food each day, too. At a minimum, aim to consume it at least three times a week.

Fermented vegetables are an excellent source of beneficial bacteria. At Mercola.com headquarters, we always have fermented vegetables on hand in the staff lunchroom. (See box on page 166 for the recipe.) And unlike some other fermented foods, they tend to be palatable, if not downright delicious, to most people. They can also be a great source of vitamin K_2 *if* you ferment your own using the proper starter culture.[23]

You could eat fermented veggies as a side dish, but I recommend adding them to a salad. They are a great substitute for vinegar, as the lactic acid in the veggies is really similar to acetic acid in vinegar. Just start out with about a teaspoonful for a few days and work your way up slowly to a few tablespoons a day to give your body time to adjust to the beneficial microbes.

Spending a portion of a weekend afternoon shredding vegetables and packing them into jars, then eating a tablespoon or so of them a few times a week, means you'll have a source of probiotics that lasts months, costs only a few dollars, and is delicious.

Most high-quality probiotic supplements will supply you with only a fraction of the beneficial bacteria found in such homemade fermented veggies, so making (and eating!) your own is your most economical route to optimal gut health as well.

When choosing fermented foods, steer clear of pasteurized versions, as pasteurization will destroy many of the naturally occurring probiotics. This *includes* most of the "probiotic" yogurts you find in nearly every grocery store these days; since they're pasteurized, they will be associated with all the problems of pasteurized milk products: heating milk, as in pasteurization, destroys a large percentage of the friendly bacteria and reduces the levels of vitamin C and vitamin B6.[24] Moreover, they typically contain added sugars, high-fructose corn syrup, artificial coloring, or artificial sweeteners, all of which will only worsen your health.

Make Your Own Food Sources of Probiotics

Fermented Vegetables

Nearly everyone who sets out to ferment vegetables is afraid they will make a mistake and create some frightful, harmful mixture. Relax, it's virtually impossible to do that; the highly acidic conditions of the fermentation kill virtually all pathogenic bacteria.

You could purchase fermented vegetables online premade, but it will likely cost you close to $20 a quart plus shipping. You can make this recipe yourself for 95 percent less.

INGREDIENTS

1 large head of organic cabbage (green or red), cored and sliced very thin or shredded in a food processor, outer leaves reserved

2 root vegetables of your choice—carrots, golden beets, radishes, or turnips—peeled and shredded in a food processor

1 or more habañero or jalapeño peppers, stem, seeds, and ribs removed and cut into a few large pieces (*Optional:* They're spicy. Leave them out if you don't like spicy. I personally use five habañeros per quart.)

1 peeled garlic clove (optional)

1 inch of peeled ginger root (optional)

1 packet of starter culture for fermenting vegetables

2 cups of fresh celery juice (or filtered water)

EQUIPMENT

1–2 quart-sized clean Mason jars

Pestle or other tool to tamp the vegetables down inside the jars

INSTRUCTIONS

Mix your prepped vegetables and the aromatics you choose (garlic or ginger) in a large mixing bowl.

In a pitcher, dissolve starter culture in freshly juiced organic celery or filtered water. You will have a higher-quality product if you use the celery juice, as it has natural sodium and potassium. Pour over the vegetables, and stir to combine.

You could ferment your vegetables without a starter culture, but the results will be far more variable, and it may take several weeks. There are a number of starter cultures on the market, but it is best to use one that has bacteria that create vitamin K_2, which is nearly as important as vitamin D.

Tightly pack the vegetable-brine mixture into each Mason jar and compress using a masher to remove any air pockets. Top with a cabbage leaf, tucking it down the sides. Make sure the veggies are completely covered with brine and that the brine is all the way to the top of the jar, to eliminate trapped air.

Put the lids on the jars *loosely,* as the contents will expand due to the gases produced in fermentation.

Allow the jars to sit in a relatively warm place for several days, ideally around 72 degrees Fahrenheit. During the summer, veggies are typically done in three or four days. In the winter, they may need seven days. The only way to tell when they're done is to open up a jar and have a taste. Once you're happy with the flavor and consistency, move the jars into your refrigerator. They will keep for many months this way, continuing to mature very slowly over time.

The vegetables are best consumed shortly after they are fermented. But they can last six months or more in the fridge, becoming mushy and losing their crunchy texture as they age.

Note: Always use a clean spoon to take out what you're eating. Never eat out of the jar, as you will contaminate the entire batch with bacteria from your mouth. Make sure the remaining veggies are covered with the brine solution before replacing the lid.

Kefir

INGREDIENTS

Milk: The highest-quality you can find—preferably raw, grass-fed (pastured), whole, and organic (exact amount will depend on the kefir-producing bacteria you use)

Kefir-producing bacteria: either powdered kefir starter culture or living kefir grains (again, exact amount will depend on which form you use; read on for more details)

EQUIPMENT

Mason jar

Stainless steel strainer

Stainless steel or ceramic bowl

INSTRUCTIONS

The exact instructions depend on whether you use a powdered culture or living kefir grains. If you are using powdered culture, you will need to gently heat the milk to about 95 degrees before combining it with the culture. (For exact ratios, follow the instructions on the packet of starter culture.)

If you are using live kefir grains, which resemble cottage cheese, you simply need to place a tablespoon of the grains in the jar and then cover with a half-cup of milk.

No matter which form of culture you use, leave the mixture out on the counter for 24 hours, or until pockets of clear liquid (whey) have begun to appear at the bottom of the jar and the milk has achieved a thick, creamy consistency. Leave the lid on loosely so your grains can breathe and so by-products of the fermentation process can escape.

If you're using a starter culture, the kefir is done at this point—you can put it in the fridge, where it will last for approximately a week.

With some cultures, you can reserve a quarter cup or so of the finished kefir to start your next batch.

If you are using a live grain, pour the mixture into the strainer that is set over a bowl. Stir the mixture to separate the finished kefir from the grains. The kefir will go into the bowl, and the grains will remain in the strainer. Pour the kefir into a glass bottle to store in the fridge until ready to drink. Rinse the grains in some fresh milk, then put back into the jar (you only need to clean this jar every few batches) and pour fresh milk in.

When using live grains, if you ever want to take a break from producing kefir every day, simply cover the grains in fresh milk in a clean jar, tighten the lid, and put them in the fridge until you're ready to start the process over again.

If Fermented Foods Aren't Appealing

Many of the people who leave comments on my site, and I myself, find fermented foods delicious and easy to make and consume. However, if they don't appeal to your palate or your to-do list, I recommend that you take a high-quality probiotic supplement. Look for one that fulfills the following criteria, to ensure quality and efficacy:

- The bacteria strains must be able to survive your stomach acid and bile, so that they reach your intestines alive in adequate numbers.
- The bacteria strains must have confirmed health-promoting features.
- The probiotic activity must be guaranteed throughout the entire production process, storage period, and shelf life of the product.

To determine if your probiotic supplement meets these criteria, check the label for the individual strains. Then look them up at Pubmed.com, a clearinghouse of peer-reviewed scientific studies that is searchable by keyword. You can visit the manufacturer's website to answer any questions you may have, or even contact the manufacturer. I know this process is not effortless, but if the probiotic supplement you take doesn't seed a population of optimal friendly bacteria in your gut, it is a waste of your money and energy, and it will leave you unprotected from the myriad benefits of a flourishing probiotic population. You only need to do your due diligence once—it's not an ongoing task.

AN EFFORTLESS PROBIOTIC AID: CHEW YOUR FOOD!

Here's a guide to ensure that you're chewing in a way that supports your health. Generally speaking, you'll want to eat in a relaxed, non-distracted environment; eating on the run or while you're working or watching TV is not conducive to proper chewing.

- Take smaller bites of food (they're easier to chew)
- Chew slowly and steadily
- Chew until your mouthful of food is liquefied or has lost all its texture
- Finish chewing and swallow completely before you take another bite of food
- Wait to drink fluids until you've swallowed

The chewing process predigests your food into small pieces and partially liquefies it, making it easier to digest. Digestion is actually a very demanding task for your body, requiring a great deal of energy, especially if it is forced to digest improperly chewed food. Chewing properly makes it easier for your gut bacteria to break down your food.

But tending to the bacteria in your gut is an ongoing process, much like tending to a flower garden. One reason is that lifestyle factors (such as stress, a course of antibiotics, or a binge of processed foods) as well as the environmental factors I discussed earlier (including chlorinated tap water, which kills gut microbes) can wipe out portions of your bacterial population.

Also, the bacteria you consume through fermented foods and probiotic supplements tend to only be visitors to your system—they live only about two weeks. When it comes to gut flora, you can't "set it and forget it." But if you provide your gut flora with the proper nourishment—fermented foods, a high-quality probiotic supplement (if you don't regularly eat fermented foods)—and avoid antibiotics and other environmental assaults, your gut bacteria will flourish and reward you exponentially in the form of good health.

| **ADVANCED EFFORTLESS HEALING** |

Fecal Transplant

One novel way to improve the makeup of bacteria in the gut sounds disgusting but is very powerful in tough cases. The fecal microbiota transplant (FMT) is proving to be incredibly effective.

The fecal transplant is actually very simple. It involves taking feces from a donor (typically a spouse or relative) and transferring it to the patient during a colonoscopy. The benefit? The patient receives a transplanted population of healthy flora that can go to work correcting any number of gastrointestinal and other health problems.

Clostridium difficile is an infection that is often resistant to antibiotics, is often debilitating, and can be fatal. According to research presented at the American College of Gastroenterology's annual meeting, fecal transplants led to the rapid resolution of symptoms in 98 percent of patients with this infection—and these patients hadn't responded to multiple previous treatments.

Separate research found that fecal transplants showed promise in the treatment of ulcerative colitis and Crohn's disease, with symptoms improving in days to weeks. Preliminary research from the Netherlands has found that transplanting fecal matter from healthy thin people into obese people with metabolic syndrome led to an improvement in insulin sensitivity.

All this research adds further credence to the immense role healthy gut bacteria can play in health.

Your Effortless Action Plan

1. *Incorporate fermented foods into your daily diet, such as yogurt or kefir made with raw milk, natto, and fermented vegetables.*

2. *Try fermenting your own vegetables. Once you experience how easy the process actually is, and how empowering it is to have an arsenal of probiotics that are delicious (and inexpensive) at the ready at all times, it will become an exhilarating piece of your good-health plan. And since you can create large amounts—enough to last months—in one shot, it will be pretty effortless!*

3. *If you don't choose to eat fermented foods at least a few times a week, seek out a high-quality probiotic supplement to take daily.*

4. *Avoid factors that harm your beneficial bacteria levels—including processed foods, sugar, antibacterial soap, and chlorinated water.*

HEALERS	HURTERS
✓ Traditionally made sauerkraut and pickles (with salt, not vinegar)	✗ Processed foods
✓ Kefir and yogurt, particularly those you make yourself (many commercial versions don't contain live probiotics, or contain a lot of added ingredients)	✗ Sugar
✓ Organic unpasteurized fermented soy, such as miso, tempeh, and natto	✗ Antibacterial soap
✓ Kombucha (a fermented beverage made from black tea)	✗ Chlorinated water
✓ Kimchee (unpasteurized)	
✓ High-quality probiotic supplements	
✓ Raw milk cheeses	

Healing Principle 7

Clean Your Brain
with Sleep

At a Glance

✓ You can eat well and exercise regularly, but if you don't sleep, your health will suffer.

✓ Sleep is an integral part of all health, particularly brain health.

✓ The hormone melatonin is a great sleep regulator.

✓ Monitoring your exposure to light normalizes your melatonin production.

✓ Sleeping pills offer too many downsides and too few upsides.

S leep is one of the great mysteries of life, like black holes and the origins of the universe. Despite mountains of sleep research, we still don't understand exactly why the body requires sleep—though we are learning more every day.

One of the most exciting functions of sleep that we are just beginning to understand is the role it plays in brain health: essentially, sleep appears to be the prime time for the brain to clear out waste products and repair itself. This new insight into sleep's role has important implications for brain health, particularly at a time when, in the United States alone, someone develops Alzheimer's every sixty-seven seconds[1]—a rate that will only increase as the baby boomers continue to age and the elderly population swells.

Why You Are Likely Not Sleeping Enough

I t's really easy to get less sleep than you need in the modern world—it's practically a badge of honor in our 24/7 society. But it's a critical mistake.

Everybody loses sleep here and there, and the body can adjust for temporary shortcomings. Life's inevitable challenges tend to disrupt sleep; cultivating good sleep habits is important to help you recover from them: like giving yourself time to wind down before bed, going to bed at the same time whenever possible, and going to bed early enough. If you have established healthy sleeping habits, it will be far easier to get back to a routine that will keep you healthy.

But even if you've read and incorporated the standard advice on good sleep habits, certain factors can work against your ability to fall and stay asleep for the recommended seven to eight hours per night. Stress, obviously, is a major influence on how well you are able to rest—lying in bed, thinking anxious thoughts, is a prescription for staying awake, as most of us have experienced.

Another crucial piece of the sleep puzzle is light. Spending hours each night watching TV, catching up on e-mails, or playing a game or viewing a movie on a mobile device are all pervasive habits that wreak havoc on the body's internal clock, known as the circadian rhythm. This clock rules the sleep-wake cycle, and when it gets out of whack, restorative sleep becomes elusive. (I'll discuss this issue in more depth in a few pages.)

Effects of Not Sleeping Enough

Why should you care about how much you sleep? You should care because not getting enough sleep can cause major health and performance issues.

Poor Memory and Concentration

You've likely experienced this one: after a poor night's sleep, you can't recall details, or you leave the house without your keys. It's no mere coincidence—significant memory impairment can occur after just a single night of poor sleep. It impairs your ability to think clearly the next day and decreases your problem-solving ability.

Heightened Stress Levels

Poor sleep can raise your levels of corticosterone, the stress hormone associated with road rage. When your body is stressed, adrenaline increases your heart rate and blood pressure, makes your muscles tense, and slows your digestive processes. Chronic high stress can lead to a variety of health problems, including:

- Headaches
- Indigestion
- Increased anxiety
- Depression
- High blood pressure

Weight Gain and Pre-Diabetes

Poor sleep can increase your risk of gaining body fat, impair your ability to lose excess pounds, and make it harder for you to maintain your ideal weight. When you're sleep deprived, leptin (a hormone that signals satiety) falls, while ghrelin (which signals hunger) rises, making you hungrier the next day.

Weakened Immune System

Poor sleep increases your chances of getting sick. In 1988, one of the first studies to establish a link between sleep and the immune response found that people who awakened more often during the first cycle of sleep tended to have lower levels of natural killer cells.[2] More recent research points to a link between the circadian clock (the natural rhythms of wakefulness and sleepiness) and the activity of certain genes that help detect and ward off bacteria and viruses.

Accelerated Aging

Poor sleep likely contributes to premature aging. It can interfere with growth hormone production, which helps you look and feel younger. Normally your pituitary gland releases HGH during deep sleep (and in response to high-intensity exercise). If you don't sleep deeply, your levels of this hormone plummet.

Advanced Tumor Growth

Poor sleep increases your likelihood of getting cancer.[3] This may be because melatonin—the hormone released by the pineal gland that helps regulate sleep (see page 182)—appears to have anticancer properties. Melatonin is thought to play a role in inhibiting the proliferation of a wide range of cancer cell types and triggering cancer cell apoptosis (self-destruction). But many habits of modern life, such as sleeping in a room with lights or next to a high-EMF clock radio or not getting enough bright-sunlight exposure in the daytime, suppress normal melatonin rhythms.

Increased Risk of Heart Disease and Dying . . . from Any Cause

Your circadian system "drives" the rhythms of biological activity in all the tissues and cells of your body. Poor sleep disrupts the master clock, which then disrupts the normal functioning of those tissues and cells. That's probably why disrupted circadian rhythms are implicated in everything from sleep impairment to weight gain, mood disorders, cardiovascular disease, and many other health issues. Researchers have found that people with chronic insomnia have a three times greater risk of dying than those who don't.

Clean Your Brain: The Link Between Sleep and Brain Health

Recent research has illuminated a key function of sleep: to clean the cells of your brain. The rest of your body is cleansed and detoxified by your lymphatic system, a series of ducts and glands that removes waste products and delivers nutrients to cells throughout your body. However, your lymphatic system does not have direct access to your brain. Your brain is a closed system, protected by the blood-brain barrier, which controls what can enter it and what cannot.

Your brain actually has its own, unique waste disposal system. Called the glymphatic system, it "piggybacks" on the blood vessels in your brain. (The "g" in "glymphatic" is a nod to *glial cells*—the brain cells that manage this system.) By pumping cerebrospinal fluid through your brain's tissues, the glymphatic system flushes the waste from your brain back into your body's circulatory system. From there, the waste eventually reaches your liver, where it is processed for elimination.

During sleep, the glymphatic system becomes ten times more active than during wakefulness. What is it doing? It appears to be taking out the trash. A 2013 study on mice showed that during sleep, brain cells are reduced in size by about 60 percent.[4] This creates more space in between the cells, giving the cerebrospinal fluid more room to flush out the debris.

One particular waste product that this study identified is removed in significantly greater quantities during sleep. That's amyloid-beta—the protein that forms the notorious plaques found in the brains of Alzheimer's patients.

This important function of sleep is still being fully studied in humans.

I hope these new insights on the role of sleep in brain health will persuade you to experiment with effortless ways to get more sleep.

How Much Sleep Is Enough?

C hronic lack of sleep *has a cumulative effect,* when it comes to disrupting your health, so you can't skimp on weekdays, thinking you'll catch up over the weekend. You need consistency.

Generally speaking, most adults need between six and eight hours of sleep every night. But according to the National Sleep Foundation, most American adults are just barely meeting this minimum, reportedly getting around six and a half hours per night during the week.[5] Even worse, it's hard for people to fully perceive all the impairments that chronic insufficient sleep causes in their waking lives. You can acclimate to the feeling of getting less sleep, but this doesn't mean you're performing at or even near your best. So be sure that you get to bed early enough so you can get the sleep you need, which will typically be in the range of six to eight hours every night.

Frequent yawning throughout the day is a dead giveaway that you need more shut-eye. If you tend to drift off whenever you sit or lie still or try to read, you need more sleep. If you have problems falling asleep, reading can be a powerful strategy to help you get to sleep at night. This is a strategy I regularly use.

Optimize Your Circadian Rhythm

The circadian rhythm, as I've said, is the twenty-four-hour body cycle determined by the master clock in the brain—a group of cells known as the suprachiasmatic nucleus that's located in the hypothalamus. Every cell and tissue of your body has its own twenty-four-hour rhythm, which is set by the master clock. The master clock synchronizes its twenty-four-hour pattern by the light-dark cycle of the sun.

Your body evolved over time to sync to natural day and night cycles. Our ancient ancestors slept at night in darkness and stayed awake in the exposure of bright daylight. But today most of us stay up late at night and use bright artificial light sources. That fools our master clocks into thinking it's day when it's actually night, and therefore it doesn't cue the sleepiness that guides you to get in bed.

You may be thinking, "We've had electric lighting for over a century—surely our biology has adapted to that change!" The reality is that such genetic adaptations usually require hundreds if not thousands of generations to adapt, not just a few.

Maintaining proper light exposure is key to ensuring that you get the sleep you require. In this way, you'll work with your body's natural rhythms, not against them, and fall and stay asleep effortlessly.

The Role of Melatonin

Melatonin, as I've mentioned, is a hormone secreted by the pineal gland. It is both tied to and helps set the body's circadian rhythm. It is released when the brain perceives dim light, and it contributes to the initiation and maintenance of sleep. In a natural environment—free of artificial light from lightbulbs, TVs, and smartphones—melatonin levels begin to rise around seven p.m. (depending on the seasons), then stay elevated until about seven a.m.

But when you have less exposure to darkness, your body produces less melatonin. Thus, exposing yourself to bright light late at night (and, interestingly, exposing yourself to insufficient bright light during the daytime) disrupts melatonin production. Just switching a bedside lamp on and off in an otherwise pitch-black room produces a drop in melatonin levels. Managing your daily exposure to light is thus a crucial piece of the sleep equation: it helps maintain proper melatonin levels.

To Sleep Better, Use Light Wisely

B efore the advent of electricity, the only light available at night was moonlight, firelight, and candlelight. All of those forms of light emit short wavelengths, which the human eye perceives as yellows, oranges, and reds. Fast-forward to now, when we not only burn lights all night but are watching TVs, using computers, and staring at all manner of gadgets.

The problem is that nearly all these kinds of light emit longer wavelengths, in the blue light spectrum.

Your body responds to wavelengths in different ways. Studies have shown that exposure to blue light at night delays the nightly peak of melatonin that triggers sleepiness, and it reduces the amount of melatonin released when the peak does come. Conversely, exposure to red light at night has a negligible impact on melatonin.[6] So if you need to use a light at night to find the bathroom, it's best to use a red light or flashlight.

If you want to protect your melatonin cycle—and maintain a consistent circadian rhythm—you should modify your environment to be more mindful of the types of light you are exposed to throughout the day. Expose yourself to bright light—which contains the longer, blue wavelengths and thus suppresses melatonin and alertness—during the day, and limit your nighttime lights to sources that emit the yellow, orange, or red portion of the light spectrum.

Here are a few powerful yet easy ways to regulate your light exposure and thus your circadian system. Establish these good habits, so you can stop wrestling with sleep and enjoy it instead.

Amp Up Your Exposure to Daytime Light

Fling open the curtains when you wake up, and fill your work-space with bright light. Go outside and enjoy the sunshine—even in the wintertime, when the sun is too low in the sky to provide vitamin D: the rays will still help set your internal clock. During winter, when light is fleeting, or when it's cloudy for days at a time, consider using blue lights intended for the treatment of seasonal affective disorder (SAD) during the day to signal to your master internal clock that it is daytime.

Use Electronics Mindfully at Night

The glow of televisions, smartphones, laptops, and handheld de-vices can all upset your circadian rhythm and promote wakeful-ness. Turn them all off at least an hour before bed.

Filter Blue Light in the Evening and Night

Aim to expose yourself to the red, yellow, and amber end of the light spectrum in the evening. Choose a digital clock with num-bers that are red instead of blue. Choose a night-light with a "low blue" lightbulb.

There are apps that filter the blue light emitted by the screens of electronic devices. If you must use these devices at night, they can reduce your exposure to blue light. Install the free utility for your computer, tablets, or phone called f.lux. The program will adjust the glow of your monitor, both the brightness and the tint, based on the time of day; it will dim your monitor or screen once it starts to get dark outside.

You can further minimize your exposure to blue light at night by wearing amber glasses. These orange-tinted glasses filter out the blue light frequencies. Ideally, you'd wear them for a few hours before going to bed.

Make Nighttime Dark

Use blackout curtains to shut out ambient light from outside. Turn digital alarm clocks away from you so the glow doesn't keep you up. Consider using a sleep mask.

Other Environmental Changes That Promote Sleep

Create a Sleep Sanctuary

Remove distractions from your bedroom—computers, TVs, etc. Make this important room a place to rest (and spend time with your partner), and your body will start to unwind as soon as you enter it.

Keep It Cool

Many people keep their homes and particularly their upstairs bedrooms too warm. Studies show that the optimal room temperature for sleep is quite cool, between 60 and 68 degrees Fahrenheit (15.5 and 20 degrees Celsius). Keeping your room cooler or hotter can lead to restless sleep.

Stay Consistent

Find yourself an easy going-to-bed routine, and stick with it as much as possible. Turn off the TV, turn down the heat, do a few minutes of stretching, brush your teeth, read (under a low-blue light). . . . It doesn't need to be complicated, it just needs to be consistent—meaning it starts at basically the same time each night.

Those of you who are parents may notice that a lot of the advice I've just listed is very similar to the advice given to new mothers and fathers to help teach their infants to sleep through the night. You and your good health deserve every bit of the attention and care you would give to a baby. Once good habits are established (more on changing behaviors in Chapter 3), they become second nature and are easy to maintain going forward.

Eat for Sleep

Promoting your circadian rhythms by monitoring your exposure to light is not the only tool at your disposal. Many nutrients also play a role in healthy sleep. And eating these nutrients in food—rather than getting them through supplements—is the most holistic way to make sure your body has the building blocks to regulate sleep. Aim to eat the following foods several times a week:

Almonds

Almonds are rich in magnesium, which is needed for quality sleep. A study published in the *Journal of Orthomolecular Medicine* found that when the body's magnesium levels are too low, it makes it harder to stay asleep. And your body is likely lacking in magnesium, as dietary surveys suggest as many as 80 percent of Americans are simply not getting enough magnesium from their diet.

Avocados

In addition to being rich in high-quality fats, avocados are an excellent source of potassium. Potassium works synergistically with magnesium to improve sleep, among other things. It's generally recommended that you take in five times more potassium than sodium.[7] But most Americans' diets are so rich in high-sodium processed foods that they consume twice as much sodium as potassium. Eating more avocados is an excellent way to bring that ratio back toward healthy levels. (Forgoing salty processed foods is another.) And the extra potassium will help your body get the sleep it needs. Green vegetable juice is also loaded with potassium.

Chamomile Tea

Drinking a cup of chamomile tea before bed is more than just a folk remedy. Researchers have found that it's associated with a rise in glycine, a chemical that has sedative properties and that promotes muscle relaxation.[8] Try drinking a cup an hour before bedtime.

Cherries

A good night's sleep is a bowl of cherries—literally, as these luscious fruits contain magnesium. Have a handful (no more) an hour before bedtime (unless you are incorporating intermittent fasting; then take them three hours before bedtime).

Green Leafy Vegetables

Greens such as kale, Swiss chard, and spinach are loaded with minerals that promote sleep. They are rich in calcium, which helps your brain use tryptophan to manufacture melatonin. And they are excellent sources of magnesium. These sleep-enhancing nutrients are yet another reason I am such a big advocate of green juice. My personal strategy is to drink a pint to a quart of fresh green vegetable juice every day. It is one of my primary sources of magnesium.

Walnuts

Walnuts benefit your sleep in two ways. They are a good source of tryptophan, an amino acid that helps your body make melatonin. And they contain their own melatonin, according to researchers at the University of Texas.[9]

Sleep-Enhancing Pills:
The Only One I Recommend

Remember that your body knows how to sleep. If you are experiencing insomnia or simply not getting enough rest, trust that the simple lifestyle and nutritional fixes I've discussed in this chapter will help normalize your circadian rhythms. And when that happens, your body will support you in effortlessly getting the rest you need.

At certain times, however, you may need a little extra help: you may be traveling between time zones, for example, or going through a stressful period in your life. During those times, the only supplement I advocate taking is melatonin.

Numerous scientific studies have shown that melatonin supplements help people fall asleep faster and stay asleep, experience less restlessness, and prevent daytime fatigue. Only a very small dose is required (typically 0.25 mg or 0.5 mg) to influence timing of circadian rhythms.[10] But those who struggle to get to sleep usually take higher doses (such as 3 mg) at bedtime.

Taking a dose of 3 mg can sometimes make you groggy the next day, so to help with sleep initiation, start with 1 mg near bedtime. If that amount doesn't get you to sleep, adjust your dose by no more than 1 mg per night until you get to 3 mg.

Why Sleeping Pills Aren't a Good Option

Sleep medications may have a legitimate role when a person is experiencing severe, crippling anxiety or when panic is impairing sleep.

But patients and doctors alike turn to them too quickly and too frequently. While it may be tempting to look for a pill to help you sleep, prescription pills help people ignore the primary issue that's impairing their sleep. In fact, using them helps a person ignore the cause of his or her sleep problems. Heartburn, diabetes, heart disease, arthritis, kidney disease, thyroid disease, and asthma can all hinder sleep. Taking a pill to "treat" the sleeplessness without addressing the reason you are awake may be analogous to turning a blind eye on a burning house: ignoring the house doesn't make it stop burning, and waiting to address the problem only sets the stage for that condition to worsen over time.

Beyond that, prescription sleeping pills don't increase sleep time by much: researchers have repeatedly shown that they extend sleep only an average of fifteen to twenty minutes. Interestingly, other studies have shown that some of these medications can induce *amnesia*, so upon waking, participants could not recall how they slept (or didn't sleep)!

Some sleep medications—including over-the-counter drugs containing Benadryl—have a long half-life, which means that they can still be stimulating sleepiness after you wake up the next morning. Not surprisingly, they're associated with cognitive deficits during the daytime. You know, like when you're likely *driving* to work.

Chronic use of sleeping pills has been linked to significant health hazards, including increased risk of cancer and death, although it is unknown if these medications are actually causing these health hazards.

How Life Feels When You're Well Rested

I magine being able to recall words, names, and details. Imagine not having to spend time every morning looking for your keys and cell phone. When you are rested, your immune system works better, so the tickle in your throat that you occasionally feel won't develop into a full-blown cold, and you won't lose days to congestion, coughs, and general discomfort. When your body can support you properly, it will make so many areas of the rest of your life feel effortless in comparison to how they feel when you're dragging yourself around after not enough sleep.

| ADVANCED EFFORTLESS HEALING |
Track Behavior to Stay Mindful

I am a big fan of tracking health and behavior, which is why I love tools such as the ones made by Fitbit. You can wear these products like a wristwatch to effortlessly collect data about how you're living. The data can be easily transmitted to various Web-based services and apps to make your personal health data even more interesting and useful!

For example, Dr. Dan Pardi is a sleep researcher who developed Dan's Plan (dansplan.com). The tool guides you to set goals for things like weight, sleep, and activity. It records and integrates data from a large number of devices (so choose the one you want to use). It then helps you stay on track to meet your daily to weekly health goals for healthy living—in your Zone of Health™. Having this sort of feedback is proven to help stimulate positive health behaviors. These new devices and services are an excellent complement to living healthfully.

Your Effortless Action Plan

1. Expose yourself to bright light during the day: sunshine, full-spectrum lightbulbs, and even blue lights intended to treat SAD during winter or perpetually cloudy weather.

2. Use "low blue" bulbs for night-lights and bedtime reading lamps, and use a digital clock with red numbers instead of blue ones.

3. Eliminate sources of nighttime light in your bedroom.

4. Establish a simple wind-down routine to prepare yourself for bed each night.

5. Keep your bedroom between 60 and 68 degrees at night.

6. Integrate a sleep-tracking device, such as Fitbit, with Dan's Plan to keep you mindful of your daily sleep practice.

7. Prioritize eating foods that promote sleep, including greens, avocados, walnuts, almonds, cherries, and chamomile tea.

8. Consider using melatonin supplements to reduce jet lag or to facilitate better sleep and a consistent circadian rhythm.

HEALERS	HURTERS
✓ Bright light during the day	✗ Dim lights during the day, or lack of access to sunshine outdoors or through windows
✓ Exposure to only amber light after the sun goes down	✗ Exposure to blue light in the evening or night
✓ Choosing and sticking to a consistent bedtime	✗ Varying when you go to bed each night
✓ Blackout curtains and sleep masks	✗ Night-lights
✓ "Low blue" lightbulbs in your bedside table lamps	✗ Using electronic devices in the hour before bed
✓ Alarm clocks with red numbers	✗ Alarm clocks with blue or green numbers
✓ Taking time to wind down before bed	✗ Working or watching TV right up until the time you get in bed
✓ Green leafy vegetables (including green juice)	✗ Sleeping pills (except in a few extreme cases)
✓ Chamomile tea	
✓ Avocados	
✓ Almonds and walnuts	

Healing Principle 8

Go Barefoot—and Other Ways to Stay Grounded

At a Glance

✓ Walking barefoot outside not only feels great, it improves your health, primarily by reducing inflammation and making your blood flow more easily.

✓ Touch is an important part of health—hugging, kissing, and (safe) sex play a significant role in your Effortless Healing plan.

✓ Laughter has numerous physical and emotional benefits. It can help even big changes feel more effortless.

✓ Breathing correctly, through your nose, is energizing and helps your body get the oxygen it needs to fuel Effortless Healing.

✓ When other means of getting grounded don't work to improve your emotional health, the Emotional Freedom Technique can provide lasting changes in a minimal amount of time.

If you've read this far, you may be thinking that while Effortless Healing may in fact be possible, it's not a whole lot of fun. I understand that weaning yourself off sugar, or pushing yourself to your maximum while exercising, may not make you want to jump up and down with joy. But take heart—Effortless Healing offers just as many healthy habits that are rewarding, enjoyable, and feel great for everyone.

All the techniques in this chapter intrinsically feel good. Laughing, kissing, hugging, breathing, and walking barefoot in the grass are some of life's simple pleasures. But these activities provide much more than a nice experience. They help you connect to something outside yourself: in layman's terms, they are grounding. When your thoughts or emotions are swirling inside your head, the practices I'm about to outline all help calm you, shift your focus away from your stressors, and provide powerful physiological benefits to boot.

A Light Touch

A truly effortless way to improve your health is to touch and be touched more. You could eat only the most wholesome foods, and stay active throughout the day, and still you would not thrive if you were not in regular physical contact with other humans.

Making skin-on-skin contact with another person—think hugging, kissing, and yes, having sex—boosts you physically and emotionally. While many factors contribute to these health benefits, one of the most important is oxytocin, aka "the love hormone."

Physical touch triggers the pituitary gland to release oxytocin, a neuropeptide. Women in childbirth release oxytocin—it helps them turn their focus away from the pain and gets them ready to bond with the baby. Men release it when they have an orgasm. So oxytocin is a key factor in life-giving events.

Even if you aren't in the throes of labor or lovemaking, oxytocin has many powerful benefits to impart. Primarily, it soothes the stress response, by counteracting cortisol (a hormone released in response to stress) and lowering blood pressure. Oxytocin also lessens the increase in heart rate that typically follows a stressful event.[1]

Oxytocin has been found to reduce people's cravings for drugs,[2] alcohol,[3] and even sweets.[4] It helps reduce excessive inflammation[5] and promotes wound healing.[6] Emotionally, it helps you feel bonded to another person, which keeps feelings of isolation and detachment at bay. It is likely a main reason pet owners recover more quickly from illness; why members of couples live longer than single people; and why support groups are so effective for people with chronic diseases and addictions.

The benefits of oxytocin that we are already aware of are plenty powerful, but there are likely just as many that are still to be uncovered. For your emotional and physical health, make warm, intimate relationships a priority, no matter what stage of life you are in. It's an important ingredient of both emotional and physical health.

The Importance of Hugs

One of the simplest ways to raise your levels of oxytocin and receive its stress-reducing and soul-soothing benefits is to hug more. Longer hugs—at least twenty seconds—appear to be better at significantly improving oxytocin levels, but any hug of any duration between two willing huggers is better than no hugs at all.

Hug your friends when you see them, snuggle up to your partner and ask for a hug, and hug your kids before they head off to school and when they come home at the end of the day.

If hugging people more doesn't feel effortless to you, hug and snuggle your pet. Just a few minutes of petting your dog or cat can trigger the release of oxytocin.

What's in a Kiss?

Another powerful form of touch is kissing. This uniquely human habit is said to have evolved as a way of sharing germs and building immunity. But that's not very romantic, is it? Clearly, there's more to a kiss than that, otherwise we wouldn't on average spend 20,000 minutes of our lives doing it.[7]

The health benefits of kissing are numerous. Researchers at Arizona State University found that couples who prioritized kissing more for a period of six weeks reported significant reductions in their stress levels, greater relationship satisfaction, and improvements in their total cholesterol levels.[8] Kissing has also been shown to boost the immune system[9] and reduce allergic responses in people with skin or nasal allergies.[10] These benefits happen in addition to the release of oxytocin that kissing also prompts.

The Joy of Sex

No list of healing forms of touch would be complete without a few notes about sex.

In just one lovemaking session, you burn calories, increase your heart rate, and strengthen muscles, making it an effective form of exercise. You release hormones that can reduce pain from menstrual cramps, arthritis, and headaches. And you release oxytocin, which, in addition to the benefits I've already mentioned, also promotes restful sleep.

When you have sex regularly over time, you can enjoy

additional benefits. People who have sex once or twice a week have significantly higher levels of immunoglobulin A (IgA), which is the immune system's first responder. IgA fights off invaders at their entry points; healthy levels of it can mean that the rest of your immune system doesn't even need to get involved. Men who have sex at least twice a week are 45 percent less likely to develop cardiovascular disease than men who do it once a month or less.[11]

And the oxytocin you release during sex also helps you feel more bonded to your partner, which provides emotional stability. As long as you're engaging in safe sex practices, increasing your sexual activity is a surefire path to better health!

If Your Sex Life Has Fizzled

Psychological forces can take a heavy toll on libido for both men and women. It's all too easy to get stuck in feeling too stressed for sex, which then only perpetuates that amped-up feeling, as sex is a great stress reliever.

All the Healing Principles I've discussed up to now will help your sex life, too. Recalibrating your blood sugar levels and your receptivity to insulin and leptin will support your libido; high levels of blood sugar turn off the gene that regulates your sex hormones.[12] If sex feels like too big a problem to tackle, prioritizing more simple touch, such as hugs and kisses, will help your bond with your partner grow—thanks to oxytocin—and make you both more in the mood. And if troublesome emotions are a big presence in your love life, the Emotional Freedom Technique I'll discuss a little later in the chapter can help release and rewire those feelings and thoughts.

Laugh It Off

Keeping a positive outlook and finding ways to stay light-hearted are invaluable parts of your journey to Effortless Healing. And one of the best ways to do both is to laugh.

Laughter can be thought of as a vigorous workout. In fact, researchers at the University of Maryland found that it promotes vasodilation—the ability of the blood vessels to expand—along with a fifteen-minute bout of exercise.[13] This makes laughter great for your health, as poor vasodilation is a risk factor for heart attack and stroke.

Other studies have found that laughter raises levels of endorphins—the feel-good hormones that boost mood and reduce pain. And Japanese researchers found that type 2 diabetics who watched a funny show while eating a meal had significantly smaller spikes in blood sugar than those who listened to a boring lecture.[14]

In a study of patients allergic to dust mites and other common irritants, patients' skin lesions shrank after they watched Charlie Chaplin's antics in *Modern Times,* whereas watching a video containing weather information had no effect.[15]

Other recorded benefits of laughing include:

- Relaxation and decreased muscle tension
- Lowered stress hormone levels
- Reduced blood pressure
- Increased levels of IgA
- Lessened perception of pain

Luckily, the Internet is a rich source of humorous videos (goats screaming like humans, anyone?) that will help you reap all these benefits for yourself. Watching your favorite funny shows or

THE CONNECTION BETWEEN
FAITH AND HEALTH

No discussion of ways to improve health by staying connected to the outside world would be complete without addressing faith. Once upon a time meditation was seen as something esoteric, but researchers are now heralding it as a powerful health tool; similarly today, spirituality and prayer will certainly become a bigger focus of the medical community in the not-too-distant future. In 1995 only three of the 125 medical schools in the United States offered courses that explored the connection between spirituality and health; but in 2013 over 90 medical schools did.[16]

Science is beginning to catch on to the powerful intersection of spirituality, the mind, and medicine—three realms that native cultures have long revered as inseparable. In 2012 researchers at McLean Hospital, a psychiatric institution affiliated with Harvard Medical School, asked 159 patients with prominent symptoms of depression how strongly they believed in a god.[17] The patients' symptoms were assessed when admitted and again upon release from the program.

Those whose belief in a god was stronger were twice as likely to respond well to the treatment. They experienced significantly better outcomes, such as:

- Lessened depression
- Reduced self-harm
- Increased psychological well-being (peace of mind, ability to have fun, general satisfaction)

Numerous studies have also found that subjects who either attended religious services regularly or considered themselves to be spiritual live longer and take better care of themselves.[18] Advice on how to strengthen your connection to a higher power falls beyond the scope of this book. Just know that any way you feel called to deepen your spirituality will likely ease your soul, your mind, and your body.

movies is actually a great use of your time, since when you laugh, you're helping yourself stay positive. The more opportunities you give yourself to laugh, the more you'll attract others who are also upbeat. Together you'll inspire each other to keep a light heart, even when you're tackling changes that seem hard at first.

Breathe Right, Now

Getting oxygen into your cells is every bit as important as eating the right foods and drinking fresh, pure water. But we usually take breathing for granted, in spite of it being our most fundamental need.

Your life likely is far removed from that of your ancient ancestors. Thanks to technology and economic improvements, you are more comfortable, with improved living standards and sanitation. But you are also susceptible to the damage caused by consumption of processed foods, competitive stress in school and at work, and far less physical exercise. All these factors negatively influence your breathing.

You may not realize it, but carbon dioxide plays an essential role in utilizing the oxygen within your body. When your carbon dioxide level is too low, changes in your blood pH make your red blood cells (hemoglobin) less able to release oxygen to your cells.[19] This is a problem because oxygen is the fuel for your cells. Without enough oxygen, your cells can't perform their duties optimally—they become more susceptible to viruses, and they can't create as much energy.

The first step to radically improving your breathing—and thus your levels of carbon dioxide and oxygen—is to breathe exclusively through your nose. Your respiratory system is not designed for you to breathe constantly through the mouth. Mouth breathing results in many common complaints and health issues such as difficulty sleeping, low energy, weight gain, headaches, dehy-dration, and even low libido. Luckily, it is very simple to gradu-ally transition back to nose breathing day and night. The Buteyko breathing method, named after the Russian physician who devel-oped it back in the 1950s, is a set of easy techniques that you can incorporate into your daily routine, to get back to nose breathing.

Test Your Breathing Capacity

Buteyko breathing can help restore your normal breathing pattern, thereby improving the delivery of oxygen through-out your body. Before you get started with this powerful method, it's important to first assess the current quality of your breathing.

Dr. Buteyko developed the following simple self-test for eval-uating the quality of your breathing. You can use a stopwatch or simply count the number of seconds.

Here is the process:

1. Sit straight without crossing your legs, and breathe com-fortably and steadily through your nose.
2. Take a small, silent breath in and out through your nose. After exhaling, pinch your nose to keep air from entering.
3. Start your stopwatch (or begin counting), and hold your breath until you feel the first definite desire to breathe. On a scale of 1 to 10, the urgency to breathe would be a 6 or a 7. It may come in the form of involuntary move-ments of your breathing muscles, or your tummy may jerk, or your throat may contract.
4. When you feel the first distinct urge to take in air, resume breathing and note the time.
5. Your inhalation after the breath hold should be calm, con-trolled, and through your nose. If you feel the need to take in a big breath, then you held your breath too long.

The time you just measured, called the control pause (CP), reflects your body's levels of carbon dioxide. A short CP time correlates with chronically depleted CO_2 levels. Every five-second increase in your CP will bring greater energy throughout the day and improved endurance during exercise. Here are the criteria for evaluating your CP result:

- **40 to 60 seconds:** Indicates a normal, healthy breathing pattern and excellent physical endurance
- **20 to 40 seconds:** Indicates mild breathing impairment, moderate tolerance to physical exercise, and potential for health problems in the future (most people fall into this category)
- **10 to 20 seconds:** Indicates significant breathing impairment and poor tolerance to physical exercise; nasal breathing training and lifestyle modifications are recommended (potential areas for concern include poor diet, excess stress, excess alcohol, etc.)
- **Less than 10 seconds:** Indicates serious breathing impairment, very poor exercise tolerance, and chronic health problems; consult a Buteyko practitioner for assistance

An Exercise to Improve Your Breathing

This simple exercise can help you retrain your breathing:

- Sit up straight, and place one hand on your chest and one hand on your tummy. Spend a minute or so breathing normally. Observe your inhalation and exhalation.
- As you observe your breath, apply gentle pressure to your chest and tummy with your hands. You want to create a

slight resistance that slows down your breathing so that you breathe less than you did before you began.

- You know you are doing it correctly when you feel a tolerable need for air, similar to what you would feel if you went for a brisk walk.
- Try to continue breathing in this way—feeling an increased, yet tolerable, need for air—for three to five minutes.
- If your breathing rate gets faster or your body feels tense, stop the exercise for half a minute. Return to it when your breathing has calmed.
- Two or three minutes into the exercise, you may notice an increase in the temperature of your hands or other body parts. Your nose may have become clearer, and your mouth may be producing more saliva. These immediate effects are due to the slight accumulation of carbon dioxide in your blood, which opens your blood vessels and airways and activates the relaxation response. Ironically, to improve blood flow and body oxygenation, we need to breathe less, not more.

Breathing through your nose during the day will help your body effortlessly find its balance between oxygen and carbon dioxide. And by practicing the above technique, you'll teach yourself how to breathe more efficiently, so that even when you are exerting yourself, you'll be able to maintain breathing through your nose and won't feel the need to gulp air through your mouth.

Walking Barefoot

When was the last time you kicked off your shoes and reveled in feeling the earth under your feet?

Has it been a while?

It may sound hard to believe, but engaging in this simple pleasure can be a powerful health-promoting activity. This startling realization is just beginning to gather scientific momentum.

A 2012 review of the research on the health benefits of connecting the human body to the ground (which is known by the terms "grounding" or "Earthing"), published in the *Journal of Environmental and Public Health*,[20] found that grounding has been shown to:

- Improve quality of sleep and feelings of restfulness upon waking
- Significantly reduce muscle stiffness and chronic pain
- Regulate the secretion of cortisol (a stress hormone) so that it adheres to a typical cycle of peaking in the morning and dipping lowest at midnight, promoting more restful sleep, regulating blood sugar levels and appetite, and contributing to weight control
- Balance the autonomic nervous system by stimulating the parasympathetic nervous system (which rules the "rest and digest" functions of the body) and quieting the sympathetic nervous system (which cues the "fight or flight" response)
- Reduce the severity of the inflammatory response after intense workouts
- Raise heart rate variability, your heart's ability to respond to stimuli and alter the pace of its beating; anytime you improve heart rate variability, you shift into health mode, as opposed to disease mode
- Thin your blood by imparting your red blood cells with a stronger negative electrical charge on their surface, improving their ability to repel each other and to flow through the tiny capillaries. This is incredibly valuable as virtually every aspect of cardiovascular disease has been correlated with

thicker, slow-flowing blood. This blood-thinning effect is so
profound that if you are taking a blood thinner, you should
consult your doctor before you start grounding regularly.
And monitor your medication dosage carefully—your doctor may be able to adjust it.[21]

How can something so simple have such profound health
benefits? Engaging in activities that intrinsically feel good are
often good for your health—like the feeling of the afternoon sun
warming your bare skin.

Walking barefoot outside, with the soles of your feet free
to mesh with the surface of the Earth, is one such case. What
makes Earthing, or grounding—walking barefoot outside—so
powerful? It creates a direct connection between your body and
the Earth, which is not only a simple pleasure but can serve to
actually make you healthier. Like getting regular sun exposure,
walking barefoot outside is an underappreciated simple foundational practice that you can easily establish.

What Does Electricity Have to Do with It?

Without electricity, you would not be alive—and not because you
wouldn't be able to watch your favorite TV program or warm your
home at night. You are a bioelectrical being, essentially a collec-
tion of electrical circuits, in which tens of trillions of cells constantly transmit and receive energy as they govern every action
you take, every physiological function you perform, and every
thought you create.

All your movements, behaviors, and actions are energized by
electricity. You are, in fact, a conductor of electricity. Your body
is made up primarily of water, after all, in which a variety of
charged ions, called electrolytes, are dissolved.

The Earth is also an electrical entity. Charged with a virtually limitless supply of electrons that come from lightning, it is essentially a supercharged battery overflowing with electrons.

When you, a bioelectrical being, directly touch the Earth—making contact between the ground and your skin, which is an excellent conductor of electricity—you absorb a steady flow of free electrons into your body, which helps create the conditions for your body to effortlessly heal itself.

And the most effortless way to make this connection is to walk barefoot outside. (There are some caveats, which I'll cover in just a moment.)

Health Benefits of Going Barefoot Outside

Grounding works to improve health on several levels, but its most important benefit is its ability to neutralize free radicals and reduce chronic inflammation.

You've heard about free radicals—most likely in an unfavorable light, as the source of oxidative stress and damage throughout the body. But as with so many traditionally deemed bad guys, like cholesterol, there's more to the story than that. Free radicals also play a role in healing. Free radicals are electron-loving particles that are important to your immune response. If you are exposed to a virus, for example, your body will send free radicals to snatch electrons from the virus molecules, thereby destroying them. They are an important part of the healing—otherwise known as the inflammatory—response.

The problem with free radicals comes when they outnumber the bad guys, such as viruses. Think of a roving pack of vigilantes inside your body: free radicals will begin attacking anything that crosses their path, including healthy cells, cell membranes, DNA, and proteins, looking for electrons to consume. Once those previously healthy cells lose an electron, they become free radicals themselves, and the process perpetuates itself. The result is an inflammatory response that is never turned off and becomes chronic. And chronic inflammation is associated with more than eighty diseases (see below for specifics).

The good news is that reconnecting to the Earth gives you access to a steady, and overlooked, supply of free electrons to neutralize free radicals when there isn't an injury to repair or an invader to combat. Grounding is the equivalent of providing your free radicals with a banquet of electrons. By quenching the fire of inflammation by neutralizing those destructive free radicals, grounding is one of the most powerful natural antioxidants you can take into your body.

DISEASES ASSOCIATED WITH INFLAMMATION

- Allergies
- ALS
- Alzheimer's disease
- Anemia
- Arthritis
- Asthma
- Autism
- Cancer
- Cardiovascular disease
- Crohn's disease
- Eczema
- Fibromyalgia
- Lupus
- Multiple sclerosis
- Pain
- Psoriasis
- Rheumatoid arthritis
- Type 1 diabetes
- Type 2 diabetes

Spending time outside with bare feet in contact with the ground even for short periods can yield significant benefits. One of my readers at Mercola.com, a schoolteacher from California, reports: "I have been sitting daily on my front porch with my feet in the grass for about thirty minutes. The first thing I noticed was that when I get up in the morning, I am not as groggy as before. I awake at six and am ready to hit the ground running. The second thing I noticed relates to digestion. Food seems to move through me at an easier pace. Now my pants fit better!"

Another reader, Graham, an artist in London, found relief from insomnia that had lasted twenty years by going barefoot in a nearby park for an hour a day. Not making any other changes, Graham was pleasantly shocked to regularly—and effortlessly—get seven and a half hours of sleep a night. He also reported waking up feeling full of energy, being more creative, and being less likely to get bogged down in minor annoyances. As an added benefit, his chronic eczema lessened dramatically and nearly disappeared. Mind you, the connection between Graham's barefoot outside time and his reduction in symptoms isn't proven. But it can't hurt you to take off your shoes when you venture outside and conditions allow.

How to Connect to the Earth

The simplest way to get grounded is to be barefoot outside with your feet directly on the Earth—whether it's dirt, sand, rock, or even an unpainted concrete sidewalk. You really start to see benefits, such as stress reduction and lessened pain, after spending thirty minutes in direct connection to the ground—but any amount of time is better than none at all. The more compromised your health is, the more time you should spend grounding. (There are a couple of exceptions, which I'll cover more in just a moment.)

That's really it—just kick off your shoes and go outside. There's no need to overthink this.

Yet you have multiple options for directly connecting to the healing energy of the Earth. Remember that some surfaces and materials are good conductors of electricity (meaning they enable electricity to flow through them) while others are insulators (meaning they prevent the flow of electricity). Also, moist surfaces are more conductive than dry ones.

Keeping all that in mind, here's a list to help you choose the best surfaces for your outdoor barefoot time. Good grounding surfaces include:

- Sand
- Grass (preferably moist)
- Bare soil
- Stone and rock
- Concrete and brick (as long as it's directly on the Earth and not painted or sealed; sealed concrete tends to look shiny and won't have small cracks running through it)[22]

The following surfaces will *not* ground you, as they are insulators:

- Asphalt
- Wood
- Rubber and plastic
- Vinyl
- Tar or tarmac

You know this innately, if you've ever done it, but because water is also an excellent conductor, an ideal location for walking barefoot is right along the water at the beach, or on grass that is wet with morning dew. (Swimming in the ocean is a fabulous way to ground, as the seawater conducts the electricity from the ocean floor. Grounding helps explain some of the renowned healing properties of saltwater.)

In order to ground, you don't have to walk, exercise, or even stand. You can sit in a chair and read a book. So long as your bare feet are in direct contact with the ground, you are officially "Earthing." You can also sit or lie on grass or sand.

Shoes

Sometimes it's simply not feasible to step outside in bare feet, either because of cold weather or because you are in an urban environment with little access to ground that isn't covered in pavement. Or perhaps work and other aspects of your life interfere with your desire to get in several minutes' worth of grounding each day. One way to maintain a connection to the Earth even when you're wearing shoes is to choose different shoes.

Synthetic rubber and plastic soles are insulators—they disconnect you from the Earth. Leather soles are conductive, meaning they permit grounding whenever you are walking on a surface that is also conductive. Although many modern shoes with leather soles have synthetic insoles and/or midsoles that make them more insulated, you can seek out traditionally made shoes with leather soles.

A growing number of companies make shoes specifically with grounding properties. A quick Internet search for "grounding shoes" or "Earthing shoes" will provide you with an ever-growing list of options. But please understand that wearing these types of soles grounds you only when you are walking on the surfaces discussed above. If you're a city dweller, don't waste your money on these shoes, unless you have access to a park or nearby beach.

Precautions

While walking barefoot is one of the simplest and most natural things you can do to improve your health, there are still some situations in which you may want to use caution, and there are even some contraindications. Remember, it isn't a treatment or a cure for anything. It simply provides "electrical nutrition" from the Earth that helps cool the inflammation associated with so many chronic diseases—an important piece of creating the conditions for Effortless Healing.

Because of the blood-thinning effects of grounding, if you are taking a prescription blood-thinner (such as Coumadin), you need to work in tandem with your doctor. In fact, individuals taking medication to thin their blood, regulate blood sugar, control blood pressure, or regulate thyroid hormone levels should consult their health care provider before doing this practice.

When you start grounding on a regular basis, your health may get worse before it gets better, depending on your health status and your toxic load. You may experience a classic detox reaction: a healing agent triggers the death of large amounts of harmful pathogens, which then release toxic by-products that make you feel sick. If you notice feeling worse after grounding, start with only ten minutes or so a day and gradually work your way up to thirty minutes. Always listen to your body to determine how much grounding feels good and appropriate to you.

Despite these caveats, grounding is an incredible, and completely natural, way to promote health—one that is available to you at virtually all times and for no or very little cost. Let your body be your guide as you decide when and how much to do it.

| ADVANCED EFFORTLESS HEALING |

Exercise Outdoors in Bare Feet

Exercising barefoot outdoors is one of the most wonderful, inexpensive, and powerful ways to incorporate Effortless Healing into your daily life. It will help you kill two birds with one stone—exercise and barefoot time. Three birds, actually, if you also expose your skin to the sun to get your daily dose of vitamin D. And barefoot outdoor exercise that's strenuous may also help speed up your tissue repair and ease muscle pain.

THE CHINESE PERSPECTIVE ON
WALKING BAREFOOT

Your skin in general is a very good conductor. Connecting any part of it to the Earth will work. But among various parts of your body, one is especially potent: a spot right in the middle of the ball of your foot. It's known to practitioners of Traditional Chinese Medicine as Kidney 1 (K1). This acupuncture point joins all the energy pathways of the body, known as meridians: that is, it connects to every nook and cranny of your body. No wonder tai chi and qigong—the Chinese equivalents to yoga—are taught and practiced outside, without shoes.

ACUPUNCTURE POINT

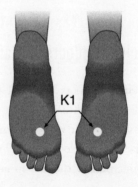

Finding Relief from Troublesome Emotions

A t some point in your journey to Effortless Healing, you may experience vexing emotions that can't be soothed by any of the grounding techniques I've covered in this chapter.

Anytime you find yourself experiencing an unpleasant feeling—such as anxiety, fear, resistance, anger, or doubt—that is impeding your ability to make healthy choices, a powerful tool can help you purge the emotion from your body and your psyche. It's literally at your fingertips, and it's called EFT (Emotional Freedom Technique).

EFT is a form of psychological acupressure—a do-it-yourself form that uses your fingertips to stimulate specific points on the body. It's based on the same energy meridians that traditional acupuncture has used to treat physical and emotional ailments for over five thousand years, but without the invasiveness of needles. Instead, you perform simple tapping with your fingertips on specific spots on your head and chest while you think about your specific problem—whether it is a traumatic event, an addiction, or a pain—and voice positive affirmations.

Tapping the energy meridians while voicing positive affirmations works to clear the "short-circuit"—the emotional block—from your body's bioenergy system, thus restoring your mind and body's balance, which is essential for disease healing and for optimal health.

If you're shaking your head in disbelief, keep reading, as you're not alone. Some people are initially wary of the principles that EFT is based on—the West has only recently begun to recognize the energetic component that has been part of other healing traditions for so long. Others are initially taken aback by (and sometimes amused by) EFT's tapping-and-affirmation methodology.

But more than any traditional or alternative method I have used or researched, EFT works to help people resolve difficult emotions once and for all. I have witnessed the results in my patients since I started using this method back in mid-2001. Indeed, because of its very high rate of success, the use of EFT has spread rapidly, and medical practitioners employing it can now be found in every corner of the country and world. If you're still skeptical, you can go to the link at the end of this section. And consider giving it a try, despite your skepticism, because what have you got to lose? Only some old thought patterns that are likely keeping you from making changes that could powerfully benefit your health and happiness.

Here are just a handful of the benefits offered by EFT:

- Relieves most emotional traumas
- Abolishes phobias and post-traumatic stress
- Shatters food cravings that sabotage your health
- Eliminates or significantly reduces most physical pain and discomfort

I have been a fan of energy psychology for many years, having witnessed its effectiveness in my own medical practice and having personally helped hundreds of patients resolve health problems with it. However, in the past, studies have been few and far between, as science has been trying to catch up with clinical experience. That has finally started to change. Several studies have been published in the last few years, showing just how safe and effective EFT really is.

For example, the following three studies found that people with a history of trauma who used EFT made remarkable progress in a very short period of time:

1. In a 2012 study published in the *Journal of Nervous and Mental Disease* (the oldest peer-reviewed psychiatry jour-

nal in the United States), subjects who received one one-hour EFT session reported a 24 percent drop in the stress hormone cortisol. The EFT group also experienced a drop in depression and anxiety that was more than twice the level experienced by subjects who had a talk therapy session or merely rested.[23]

2. A 2013 study published in the same journal studied 59 veterans diagnosed with post-traumatic stress disorder (PTSD). Participants received six EFT sessions; after six months, the reductions in depression and anxiety were still so significant that 86 percent of the veterans no longer met the clinical definition of PTSD.[24]

3. EFT has also been proven to be effective in groups as well as in individual treatment. In 2014 veterans and their spouses attended a seven-day EFT retreat. Upon arrival, 89 percent of the veterans met the criteria for PTSD, as did 29 percent of the spouses. After the retreat, only 28 percent of the veterans had PTSD, and only 4 percent of the spouses.[25]

I once gave an EFT demonstration in front of four hundred clinical nutritionists. A volunteer came up who had a severe craving for the Rice Krispies treats in the exhibit area. Her craving was a strong 10 out of 10. As soon as we did one round of tapping, she was on the verge of tears. When I explored the issue further with her, she said that she was reminded of the time when her mother would give her M&M treats to get her out of her hair.

The real issue had nothing to do with her craving for treats; instead, she was "craving" the love and attention that her mother did not give her. We tapped on that issue, and her craving for the sweets disappeared instantly.

For more information on EFT, please visit http://eft.mercola .com.

Your Effortless Action Plan

1. *Make time for touch. Kissing, hugging, and having sex all help you feel bonded to others, which is supportive of your emotional health. Touch also triggers a cascade of physiological benefits that help your body function better and more effortlessly.*

2. *Prioritize laughing. Watching funny movies and silly videos on the Internet are much more than time wasters—they are powerful health boosters.*

3. *Train yourself to breathe through your nose. Mouth breathing depletes your body of oxygen and carbon dioxide and creates a barrier to good health. The more you can breathe quietly through your nose, the healthier you will be.*

4. *Walk barefoot outside whenever possible—thirty minutes a day is recommended, but any amount is better than none.*

5. *For unpleasant emotions that may be hindering your ability to make positive changes, seek out an Emotional Freedom Technique practitioner. Although the practice is very effective when done on your own, a practitioner can help you home in on the exact phrases that will resonate with you the most, and show you how to do it correctly.*

HEALERS	HURTERS
✓ Laughing	✗ Watching only serious TV programs or movies
✓ Kissing	✗ Letting a low libido or high stress levels keep you from a healthy sex life
✓ Hugging ✓ Having (safe) sex	✗ Not taking ample opportunities to hug others; pets count
✓ Walking barefoot outside	✗ Keeping your shoes on when you're at the park or beach
✓ Breathing through your nose	✗ Breathing through your mouth
✓ Repeating affirming phrases while tapping specific points on the body with your fingertips (EFT)	✗ Not seeking a release for your troublesome emotions

Healing Principle 9

Avoid These Six "Health Foods"

At a Glance

✓ Much conventional wisdom about what is healthy is not only false, it's harmful.

✓ Stealth "health" foods that should be avoided are:

 ✗ Whole grains like brown rice

 ✗ Natural sweeteners such as agave

 ✗ Unfermented soy products, including tofu and soymilk

 ✗ Vegetable oil

 ✗ Most types of fish

 ✗ Conventional yogurt

P art of the challenge in seeking Effortless Healing is that many food marketers and often unsuspecting or unschooled members of the media will deceive you about what's in your food. When the foods they promote as being healthy actually zap your health away, it becomes a serious issue.

By constantly introducing harmful chemicals, hormones, and proteins into your body via the food you regularly eat, you hinder your body's ability to heal itself effortlessly. And when you are consuming these foods while under the belief that you are actually benefiting your body, you keep yourself trapped in a state of suboptimal health. The foods I'm about to discuss serve mostly to give your body "busy work." They force your body to strive to counteract their detrimental effects and to keep it from what it was designed to do—easily and efficiently regenerate itself.

In this chapter, I discuss the top six foods that are often heralded for their health properties but that you would be well served to avoid. I also offer alternatives for each. By swapping out the bad for the good, you'll be removing a huge burden from your body. Eliminating the offenders and replacing them with their more healthful counterparts will reward you with significantly improved energy levels, ability to shed excess pounds, and overall vitality.

Grains

O ne of my readers, Denise, is the mother of two. As she approached forty, she was thirty pounds over her ideal weight, and her blood pressure was creeping up as well. Denise had a master's degree in nutrition and had held fast to a low-fat, high-fiber diet, heavy on the whole grains, for nearly twenty years (just as I had done back in the 1970s). Every few months she would periodically embark on a diet regimen of eating 1,200 calories a day and doing cardio for five to six hours a week, only to feel hungry, grumpy, and as heavy as ever.

Denise finally got annoyed by the idea that being overweight was just "the way it is" for a forty-something woman. She agreed to give up her toast at breakfast and her sandwich at lunch and replace those grains with high-quality fat—an egg with cheese for breakfast, a handful of nuts for a snack, and salad with plenty of olive oil as a dressing for lunch. And the weight started to melt off. After two and a half years of eating low-to-no-grain and -gluten, Denise has lost and kept off thirty-five pounds. Her blood pressure is normal. And her good-to-bad-cholesterol ratio and triglyceride levels are well within healthy ranges. Perhaps best of all, Denise has been inspired to start using that master's degree to counsel patients on healthy eating—with a low-grain twist.

It's no wonder if you, like Denise, have come to mindlessly revere whole grains as superfoods. The USDA website (http://www.choosemyplate.gov/food-groups/grains-why.html) will tell you that consuming whole grains may reduce your risk of heart attack, reduce constipation, and help you control your weight.

Insulin and Leptin Resistance

The reason the across-the-board recommendation to eat more whole grains is unwise is that so many of us struggle with insulin or leptin resistance. You see, even "healthy" whole grains are carbohydrates. And carbohydrates, even those from whole grains, cause a rise in blood sugar that then triggers the release of insulin in the body.

The role of insulin is to help drive sugar from your bloodstream into your cells, where it can be used for energy. But your cells have a limited capacity to use and store sugar. So when you regularly eat excessive sugar and carbohydrates, the excess sugar gradually builds up in your blood. When this happens, your body produces even more insulin to lower the sugar in your blood, because it knows that excess sugar in your blood is harmful and that if it goes high enough, it will even kill you (as I discussed in Healing Principle 3). When your body produces more and more insulin because you are constantly eating sugars and/or grains, the insulin receptors on your cells become increasingly tolerant to insulin. This causes your body to produce even more insulin to lower your blood sugar. This vicious cycle continues over many years and is the primary reason for insulin resistance, or, more accurately, decreased sensitivity of your insulin receptors to insulin.

There are medications to treat insulin resistance. The only way to stop perpetuating it is to change your diet and to exercise. Many physicians are seriously confused about this fact and give insulin to type 2 diabetics to lower their blood sugar, which actually makes their insulin resistance worse and contributes to their premature death.

The same process occurs with leptin resistance. Leptin is a hormone made by your fat tissue that helps your brain regulate your food intake and body weight. Since the treatments for leptin and insulin resistance are identical, many experts simply refer to insulin resistance, as it is better known.

You should avoid grains if you are either insulin or leptin resistant.

How Do You Know if You Are Insulin or Leptin Resistant?

The most accurate way to know is to measure your blood insulin level. The lower your level, the better. A level below three indicates you do not have insulin resistance. As a less expensive—and more effortless—alternative to blood testing, you can assess your own symptoms.

You may well have an element of insulin or leptin resistance if you have any one of the following conditions:

- Overweight—over 10 percent of your ideal body weight
- Type 2 diabetes or a fasting blood sugar greater than 100
- High blood pressure
- Less-than-ideal cholesterol ratios
- Cancer
- Heart attack, angina, stroke, or transient ischemic attacks

If you do have one of these conditions, you're not alone. About 85 percent of the population has at least one. Insulin and leptin resistance are not the sole cause of these conditions, but they play a major role in nearly all cases. When it comes to cholesterol, the improper signaling of insulin and leptin cues LDL cholesterol (the "bad" cholesterol that accumulates inside arteries, leading to atherosclerosis and heart disease) to become smaller and denser,[1] making it more apt to squeeze into the cracks between cells in the arteries, where it then oxidizes and contributes to inflammation.

In the case of cancer, insulin encourages cell growth, and cancer is the proliferation of fast-growing cells. Although the mechanism that causes cancer's formation and its growth is complex, numerous studies have linked insulin resistance with specific types of cancer. In fact, a 2009 review of studies that included over 500,000 people found an increased risk of cancer, and of dying of cancer, for every extra unit of glucose in the blood.[2]

If you have the signs of insulin or leptin resistance, then eating grains—yes, even organic freshly stone-ground whole grains—can actually worsen your health and lead to obesity, which is in itself a predictor of chronic disease.

The link between grains and weight is this: insulin is essentially a storage hormone, evolved to put aside excess carbohydrate calories in the form of fat in case of future famine. So as your body requires more and more insulin to process grain carbohydrates, it receives more and more signals to store fat. If you eat grains three times a day—even if those grains are from so-called superfoods such as brown rice—your body is getting three distinct orders to shuttle those calories into your fat cells. Every day.

Hold on—it gets even worse. Insulin resistance also signals your body not to burn any stored fat. This makes it exceedingly difficult, if not impossible, for you to use your own stored body fat for energy. So when you are insulin/leptin resistant, the grain carbohydrates in your diet not only make you fat, they make you stay fat. It's a double whammy, and it can be lethal. (It's important to note that you can have insulin or leptin resistance even if you are not overweight. As I said, any one of the conditions listed on page 223 suggests a good probability that your body's response to insulin and/or leptin is off track.)

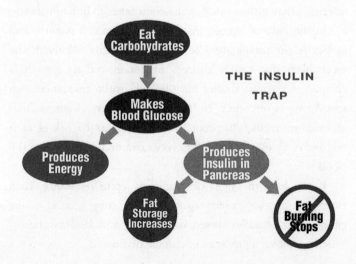

THE INSULIN TRAP

Eat Carbohydrates → Makes Blood Glucose → Produces Energy / Produces Insulin in Pancreas → Fat Storage Increases / Fat Burning Stops

The Perils of Gluten

Of course, wheat is a grain, so everything I just wrote about whole grains above pertains to the 100 percent whole wheat bread and pasta you've heard you should eat. But these faux health foods present an additional issue: gluten.

Gluten is the primary protein found in wheat, spelt, barley, and rye. By far, wheat is the most common grain that you are ingesting on a daily basis. In my experience, there is an epidemic of hidden intolerance to wheat. Most people assume that sensitivity to gluten causes only digestive problems like bloating, gas, constipation, and diarrhea, but nothing could be further from the truth. Gluten sensitivity can cause other symptoms, including strong fatigue after a meal, brain fog, dizziness, premenstrual problems, joint pain, mood swings, attention problems, and migraine headaches.

The reason is that wheat, even organic whole wheat, contains proteins such as gliadin and gluten. When these two break down into smaller proteins during the digestive process, they can find their way into your bloodstream through microscopic holes in your digestive tract. Therein lies the problem. If you are sensitive to these proteins—and up to 75 percent of the population has undiagnosed food allergies or sensitivities—your body will attack the cells that these proteins have attached to, treating those cells as a foreign invader. Your immune system is just doing its job, attacking the invader, but your organs become the collateral damage. These attacks cause toxic reactions that in turn provoke the inflammatory response.

If you eat gluten regularly, this inflammation will likely become chronic and has the potential to set off, or exacerbate, *many* other health problems throughout your body. This is why gluten can have such a devastating effect on your overall health.

Don't make the mistake of thinking you have to have the

autoimmune version of gluten sensitivity, termed celiac disease, to develop symptoms. That is not true. If you are overweight and/ or insulin or leptin resistant, I recommend that you stop eating all forms of wheat so that you eliminate gluten from your diet.

Usually when people remove allergenic foods (such as gluten) from their diet, their craving for sweets diminishes, their mood improves, their weight drops, and their overall health soars. Other benefits may include reduced joint pain, better digestion, and a clearer mind.

Once you are at a healthy weight and are free of high blood pressure, diabetes, and high cholesterol, then you can play with reintroducing grains periodically and see how well you tolerate them.

Foods to Avoid	Better Choices
Barley	Almond meal (in baking)
Millet	Buckwheat groats (steamed as a replacement to rice or ground into flour; buckwheat isn't a grain but a seed)
Oats	Buckwheat noodles (made of 100 percent buckwheat)
Rice (brown and white)	Cauliflower, either steamed and minced so as to offer an alternative to rice, or steamed and pureed with butter as an alternative to mashed potatoes
Rye	Coconut flour (in baking)
Spelt	Sweet potatoes
Sprouted grains	
Wheat	

The foods on the second list are preferable to grains, as they don't have quite the same impact on blood sugar as grains. But if you are truly insulin resistant, eating these foods regularly will slow your journey to Effortless Healing dramatically—it may take two to three times as long to heal your body's ability to process insulin and leptin. If you are insulin and/or leptin resistant, I encourage you to minimize all starchy foods so you can reap the benefits of Effortless Healing faster.

Once any of the clinical signs of insulin resistance listed above are gone, you can relax your carbohydrate restriction. At that point you can gradually reintroduce more carbs, fruits, and nongluten grains and decrease your fat. It would be wise to keep your protein level about the same and continue to avoid sugars and processed foods. Carefully monitor your weight—if it starts to climb back up, then consider resuming your original dietary plan.

Natural Sweeteners: Say Goodbye to Agave

A popular phrase on food packages and beverage bottles these days is "naturally sweetened." It implies that the foods contained within are healthier than those sweetened with regular refined sugar or artificial sweeteners. But are they?

First, a word about artificial sweeteners. Don't use them. If you have ever been to my website, Mercola.com, you already know how adamantly opposed to them I am. The many dangers of sweeteners, particularly aspartame, are so well documented that I could fill an entire book on them. (In fact, I did—it's called *Sweet Deception*.) If you're interested in more information, go to Mercola.com and type in *aspartame* in the search box at the top of every page; you'll be able to navigate to my many articles on the subject.

When it comes to so-called natural sugars, it's important to understand that there are different forms of sugar. Regular table sugar is actually composed of two simple sugars, glucose and fructose, in equal amounts. Compelling research shows that higher levels of fructose, especially if processed, are far more dangerous than glucose.

Several studies have shown that fructose has an appetite-stimulating effect that glucose doesn't have.[3] It reduces leptin (an appetite-suppressing hormone) and has no effect on ghrelin (the hunger hormone that is typically suppressed after eating). Glucose has the opposite effect—it increases leptin and reduces ghrelin. As a result, fructose appears to signal your body to eat more and to need increasing amounts of calories to feel full.

The other trouble with fructose is its relationship to fat. First, it increases triglycerides—fats stored in the blood that are associated with cardiovascular disease and stroke. It also plays an important role in how fats are processed and stored in your body.

Every cell in your body can use glucose (and also dextrose, which is another name for glucose), but only your liver can metabolize fructose. When your body has excess fructose, it must store the sugar as fat. And the type of fat it results in is visceral fat, which packs in and around the abdominal organs and is a major risk factor for heart disease. In many ways, excessive fructose consumption has similar repercussions to excessive alcohol consumption: both result in harmful levels of fats being stored in your liver.

Natural sweeteners such as honey and agave may seem like a healthier choice than refined sugars, but they are loaded with far higher levels of fructose. Fructose isn't a great source of calories for anyone, no matter how healthy you are. But if you struggle with insulin or leptin resistance, it can be a serious problem because of its tendency to increase appetite and visceral fat.

Agave syrup has been touted as a health food, but it has more fructose than any commercial sweetener, ranging from 70 to 97 percent depending on the brand. High-fructose corn syrup, in comparison, averages 55 percent fructose. What's worse, most agave "nectar" or "syrup" is nothing more than lab-generated supercondensed fructose syrup, devoid of virtually all nutrient value.

Honey is also high in fructose, averaging around 53 percent, but contrary to agave, it is completely natural in its raw form. It has many health benefits when used in moderation (one or two teaspoons per day—each teaspoon contains four grams of fructose) so long as you don't have any signs of insulin or leptin resistance. But you're not likely to find high-quality raw honey in your local grocery store. You would need to buy it from a local beekeeper, a health food store, or online.

> **Raw, locally grown honey may help with hay fever and other seasonal allergies.**

As a standard recommendation, I advise *keeping your TOTAL fructose consumption—primarily from fruit—below 25 grams per day*. If you drink beverages other than water and eat processed food, it would be wise to limit your fructose from fruit to *15 grams or less*, as you're virtually guaranteed to consume "hidden" fructose in these types of products.

Fifteen grams of fructose is not much—it represents two bananas, one-third cup of raisins, or two Medjool dates. Remember, the average 12-ounce can of soda contains 40 grams of sugar, at least half of which is fructose; one can of soda alone would exceed your daily allotment.

Better Sugar Alternatives

I realize that to completely remove all forms of sweetness from your diet is not quite effortless. While I do believe that the less sugar you eat, in all its forms, the healthier you will be (especially if you are insulin or leptin resistant), life sometimes requires a touch of sweetness. Here then are alternatives that don't exact a high toll on your health.

Sugar Alcohols

Sugar alcohols can be identified by the *ol* at the end of their name, such as xylitol, glucitol, sorbitol, maltitol, mannitol, glycerol, and lactitol. They're not alcohol and they are not sugar but sort of a hybrid of the two. They are frequently used as a sugar substitute but are not as sweet as sugar. They contain fewer calories, but they're not calorie-free. So don't get confused by the "sugar-free" label sometimes on foods containing these sweeteners. As with all packaged foods, you need to carefully read the food labels for calorie and carbohydrate content, regardless of any claims that the food is sugar-free or low-sugar.

In moderation, some sugar alcohols can be a better choice than highly refined sugar, fructose, or artificial sweeteners. Of the various sugar alcohols, xylitol is one of the best. When it is pure, the potential side effects are minimal, and it actually comes with some benefits, such as fighting tooth decay. All in all, I would say that xylitol is reasonably safe and potentially even a mildly beneficial sweetener. (As a side note, *xylitol is toxic to dogs* and some other animals, so be sure to keep it out of reach of your family pets.)

Sweeteners to Avoid	Better Choices
Agave	Dextrose (another name for glucose)
Aspartame	Lo han kuo (also known as lo han guo, lo han, and monk fruit)
Beet sugar	Raw local honey (no more than a teaspoon or two a day)
Brown rice syrup	Stevia (whole leaf extract in liquid or powdered form)
Brown sugar	Xylitol
Cane sugar	
Coconut sugar	
Date sugar	
Fruit juice	
High-fructose corn syrup	
Maple syrup	
Molasses	
Sorghum	
Splenda	
Sucanat	
Sucralose	
Truvia	
Turbinado	

Stevia and Lo Han

Two of the best sugar substitutes are from the plant kingdom: stevia and lo han guo (also spelled "luo han kuo" and also known as lo han or monk fruit). Stevia, a highly sweet herb derived from the leaf of the South American stevia plant, is sold as a supplement. It's completely safe in its natural form and can be used—either as a liquid or as powdered crystals—to sweeten most any recipe or drink where you would typically use sugar. It's a far safer way to give yourself a treat and really does deliver on some of the failed promises of artificial sweeteners. Lo han is a Chinese fruit, but it's a bit more expensive and harder to find than stevia. Both options are significantly sweeter than sugar, so use a very light touch when using them to sweeten food or beverages.

Watch out for the sugar substitute Truvia, which claims to be the same as stevia but makes use only of the active ingredient and not the entire plant. It also uses the sugar alcohol erythritol as the primary sweetener. Erythritol is not as safe a sweetener as stevia, as it can cause diarrhea, headaches, and stomachaches.

Soy Trouble

The vegetarian and health-food world has heralded tofu as a healthy alternative to meat, and soymilk as a substitute for cow's milk. But soy is not the healthy item many still believe it to be.

If you were to carefully review the thousands of studies published on soy, I strongly believe you would reach the same conclusion I have—which is that the risks of consuming *unfermented* soy products *far* outweigh any possible benefits.

There are four main reasons you should avoid eating unfermented soy:

- Nearly all conventional soybeans grown in the United States—91 percent—are genetically modified. And the primary genetic modification that soybeans undergo is to make them immune to the toxic pesticide Roundup. So soy crops are doused in the stuff.
- Unfermented soy contains goitrogens, substances that

hinder thyroid function. When the thyroid is suppressed, a host of health problems result, including digestive problems, food allergies, difficulty losing weight, anxiety and mood swings, insomnia, difficulty conceiving children, and many more.

• Unfermented soy contains the plant form of estrogen, known as phytoestrogen. The plant estrogens in soy have been linked to breast cancer,[4] kidney stones,[5] and impaired memory in an elderly population.[6]

• Unfermented soy contains phytates, which prevent the absorption of minerals in the body and create a deficiency.

SOY SHAKES: A NOT-SO-HEALTHY ROUTINE

An example of how the wrong type of soy can ruin your life comes from one of my subscribers, Donna, who lives in New York. She was in her mid-fifties and had consumed soy protein drinks daily for twenty years because she believed they were good for her. After twenty years of this "healthy" routine, Donna's thyroid became seriously damaged, and she wound up gaining sixty pounds. Once she read my newsletter and learned that the soy protein could be causing the problem, she stopped the protein drink.

She found a doctor who put her on a natural thyroid replacement supplement (such as Nature-Throid). Unlike most commonly prescribed thyroid hormones that provide only one form of thyroid hormone—such as Synthroid (T4) or Cytomel (T3)—desiccated thyroid hormones are taken from an animal's thyroid gland and contain all forms of thyroid hormones (T1, D2, T2, T, T3, and T4). This combination provides a more complete set of tools for the thyroid to stabilize itself and the body's metabolism.

She felt much better and she was finally able to lose those sixty pounds.

When Soy Is Healthy

I want to be clear that I am not opposed to *all* soy. It can be incredibly healthful: you may have heard that Japanese people live longer and have lower rates of cancer than Americans because they eat so much soy. But it's primarily *fermented soy* that they consume, and it's always been that way—and that is the crucial difference between their soy consumption and the typical American's.

The fermentation process effectively addresses many of the problems I just listed with unfermented soy. The long fermentation process reduces the phytate and "anti-nutrient" levels of soybeans, making their beneficial properties more available to the digestive system. In addition, fermentation dramatically reduces the levels of phytoestrogens[7] and increases the beans' protein content.[8] Fermented soy is also an excellent source of vitamin K,[9] which plays an essential role in preventing osteoporosis,[10] cardiovascular disease,[11] and dementia.[12] Vitamin K also protects you from prostate,[13] lung,[14] and liver cancer,[15] and it works synergistically with vitamin D to keep you and your bones healthy.

Fermented soy products are the only ones I recommend consuming. They include:

- **Tempeh,** a fermented soybean cake with a firm texture and nutty, mushroom-like flavor
- **Miso,** a fermented soybean paste with a salty, buttery texture (commonly used in miso soup)
- **Natto,** fermented soybeans with a sticky texture and strong, cheeselike flavor
- **Soy sauce,** which is traditionally made by fermenting soybeans, salt, and enzymes. Be wary because many varieties on the market today are made artificially, using a chemical process, and contain high levels of wheat and, therefore,

gluten. To choose a healthy soy sauce, look for an organic, gluten-free tamari. It doesn't include wheat and is fermented using traditional methods.

In addition, it is crucial that the fermented soy products that you choose be organic, because anything bearing the USDA Organic Seal is prohibited from using genetically modified products. Opting for organic miso, for example, is the only way to avoid GMOs in your soy products.

Soy Foods to Avoid	Better Choices
Edamame	Miso
Soy burgers	Natto
Soymilk	Tamari
Textured soy protein	Tempeh
Tofu	

Vegetable Oils

Vegetable oils—such as corn, soy, canola, sunflower, and safflower oils—are some of the most misunderstood and overrecommended foods in the health community. They are supposed to improve your heart health, but the evidence shows they actually increase your risk of heart disease and cancer. That's not very health promoting!

You may not purchase these oils in the grocery store directly, but if you purchase processed foods, as 95 percent of Americans do, you are getting these oils—processed foods are typically loaded with them. And worse, the highly processed industrialization of most food oils makes them even more toxic.

One of the primary problems with all oils derived from

vegetable seeds is that they are major sources of omega-6 fats. Omega-6 fats are pro-inflammatory and contribute to insulin and leptin resistance, altering your mood and impairing learning and cell repair. And Americans are eating far too many of them and not nearly enough of their healthier counterparts, omega-3 fats.

Omega-3 fats are present in fish and krill oil, in walnuts, in grass-fed beef and dairy, and in some seeds like flax, chia, and hemp. These fatty acids improve your cells' response to insulin, neurotransmitters, and other messengers, and they reduce your risk of heart disease,[16] cancer,[17] stroke,[18] Alzheimer's,[19] arthritis,[20] and a host of autoimmune diseases.[21] The main way omega-3 fats work to improve your health is by reducing inflammation throughout the body, especially in your blood vessels, and helping to optimize your cholesterol ratios, thereby reducing your risk of heart disease. The ideal ratio of omega-3 to omega-6 fats likely ranges from 1:1 to 1:5, but the typical Western diet is between 1:20 and 1:50.

Both omega-3 and omega-6 fats are polyunsaturated fatty acids (PUFAs), and they are essential to good health. But when omega-6 fats are consumed *in excess,* they become problematic. PUFAs are chemically very unstable and highly susceptible to being altered and denatured by what's around them. When you eat too many PUFAs, they are increasingly incorporated into your cell membranes. *Because these fats are unstable, your cells become fragile and prone to oxidation,* meaning the building blocks of your body become damaged. This leads to all sorts of health problems, such as chronic inflammation and atherosclerosis. For this reason, reducing your intake of omega-6 fats and balancing your omega-3:omega-6 ratios is vitally important to creating the internal conditions for your body to heal itself effortlessly.

You really don't need much omega-3 or omega-6, but if you

HOW TO RESIST JUNK FOOD

The first step to avoiding processed junk food is to change your mindset. Rather than looking at junk food as a reward that tastes good, or at its elimination as a punishment or deprivation of fun—neither of which is true—try thinking of it as:

- Extra calories that will harm your body

- A toxic concoction of foreign chemicals and artificial flavors that will lead to disease

- A waste of your money

- Likely to lead to increased health care bills for you and your family

- Not something to give to children, whose bodies are still developing and in great need of nutrients

Flip that around, too. Instead of thinking of healthy food as boring or time-consuming, as restrictive or not tasting good—again, not true—view it as fuel that will fortify your body with nutrients, boost your immune system, and fight disease—even slow down the aging process and make you feel more alive. Taking care of the bodies we live in bears huge rewards. I can't think of a stronger advertisement than that!

eat processed foods and/or cook with corn, soy, safflower, or sunflower oil, you are likely consuming *way* too much omega-6. The simplest way to bring your PUFA consumption back to healthy levels is to avoid all processed vegetable oils and replace them with the list of healthy oils on page 239.

In addition, you must consciously consume omega-3 fats, which I'll discuss how to do in just a moment. (It's not as simple as eating salmon a few times a week, as many sources of health information suggest.)

A Much-Demonized Kind of Fat

You might be surprised that among the oils I recommend are butter and coconut oil, as they are relatively high in saturated fats. For the past sixty years, conventional medical authorities have warned you to avoid saturated fat: that saturated animal fats cause heart disease and should be severely restricted in a heart-healthy diet.

This myth grew from a flawed study published over half a century ago. It's virtually impossible to estimate how many people have been prematurely killed by its persistent promulgation. Most of the studies that supported the claim that they were dangerous failed to properly control for trans fats and other dietary variables that were far more likely to cause problems. Trans fats are so bad that the FDA is now in the process of removing their "generally recognized as safe" (GRAS) status and they will most likely be banned from the food supply.

But saturated fats are not the root of all evil—and are *not* to blame for the modern disease epidemics facing Americans. On the contrary, they are incredibly healthy, nourishing, all-natural fats that humans have been thriving on for generations. Many decades of subsequently published research have soundly debunked the myth.[22]

Saturated fatty acids constitute at least 50 percent of cell membranes. They are what give cells necessary stiffness and integrity. They play a vital role in bone health. They lower Lp(a), a substance in your blood that indicates your proneness to heart disease. They protect your liver from alcohol and other toxins, such as Tylenol and other drugs, and they enhance your immune system.

Many prominent physicians still strongly discourage saturated fats, but fortunately the conventional wisdom is starting to change. So please be sure you eliminate the saturated fat nonsense-myth so you can start reaping the benefit of effortless health today.

> **Saturated fat is an important component of a diet that promotes lean body mass.**

Oils to Avoid	Better Choices
Canola oil	Avocado oil (unheated)
Corn oil	Butter (definitely organic, and pastured and raw if possible)
Hydrogenated or partially hydrogenated fats	Coconut oil (best for cooking)
Margarine	Olive oil (unheated, as it oxidizes quickly when exposed to heat)
Safflower oil	Walnut oil (unheated)
Shortening	
Soy oil	
Sunflower oil	

Large and Farmed Fish

F ish are commonly positioned as a health food, and an increasingly popular one at that. In the 1970s the average person ate 25 pounds of fish per year. It has now reached 42 pounds per person and is expected to keep rising. (By comparison, global beef consumption is at less than 20 pounds per person annually.) In 2011, for the first time in modern history, global farmed fish production topped beef production, and the gap widened in 2012 when 66 million tons of farmed fish were produced, compared with 63 million tons of beef.[23]

It is true that fish used to be one of the healthiest foods you could eat. But thanks to industrial pollution, most seafood is now contaminated with heavy metals like mercury, and chemicals like dioxin and PCBs.

Mercury is a potent neurotoxin that also damages your kidneys and lungs. More than 75 percent of your exposure to this toxin will be from eating fish. Contaminated Pacific tuna alone accounts for 40 percent of the exposure.[24]

You may wonder how the mercury got in the fish in the first place. Most of it comes from the burning of fossil fuels like coal. Since the United States burns coal to produce about 50 percent of its energy, it actually dumps 40 million tons into the air every year that eventually winds up in the ocean. Since fish are higher up the food chain, they tend to bioaccumulate and concentrate these types of toxins to much higher levels than are present in the water.

Larger fish like tuna and swordfish, which live longer and can weigh several hundred pounds, tend to have far more mercury. Smaller fish, like sardines, are lower on the food chain and tend to have far lower levels of mercury. Even the conservative EPA advises women to avoid fish particularly high in mercury, like tuna, when they are pregnant.[25] It is safe to assume that their recommendation needs to be extended to all who wish to remain healthy.

In the vast majority of cases, farmed fish is not a better option than wild. Farm-raised fish have similar levels of mercury and other contaminants. In addition, they are typically fed loads of soy, but as you now know, the vast majority of soy is genetically modified and laden with pesticides. Some farmed fish are genetically modified themselves. I cannot recommend that anyone eat farmed fish—particularly anyone who is interested in improving their health.

A major pitfall to the contaminated state of our fish population is that fatty fish are an excellent source of the vitally important omega-3 fats. Unless you have lab results in your hand that verify the purity of your salmon, I strongly suggest that you get your omega-3 fats from krill oil, as it is the safest and most cost-effective choice. I used to recommend taking fish oil or cod liver oil (and I still do in some cases), but cod have been overfished to the point of near extinction, and the oil is potentially contaminated with mercury.

But fish oils have other drawbacks, too. Most important, fish oil is highly perishable. As I've said, omega-3 fat is a PUFA, and PUFAs are unstable and prone to oxidation. Most fish oil goes rancid either on the shelf or inside your body, and it can contribute to the chronic inflammation you are seeking to squelch by taking omega-3s in the first place.

Krill oil, which is made from tiny shrimplike creatures, is superior to fish oil because it contains phospholipids, antioxidants (more than forty-seven times the levels found in fish oil!), and omega-3s bonded together in a way that keeps them safe from oxidation and that makes them easily absorbed in your body. So with krill oil, you can ensure that you're getting these incredibly healthy fats (EPA and DHA) without having to worry about oxidation issues.

Additionally, your risk of getting mercury contamination is extremely low since krill are so small, they don't have the chance to accumulate toxins before being harvested, and they grow in the relatively pristine waters of the Antarctic.

Because krill makes up the diet of whales, seals, and other marine creatures, many people are concerned that consuming krill oil is equal to "stealing" the natural food of these animals. But it is not.

Krill is actually the largest biomass on Earth. There is a very large stock of renewable krill for both natural predators and humans. In addition, krill harvesting is one of the best-regulated industries today. There is even a precautionary catch limit set to ensure that krill will not be overharvested.

Personally, I now take krill oil every day.

Fish to Avoid	Better Choices
Halibut	Anchovies
Largemouth bass	Croaker
Marlin	Haddock
Pike	Herring
Salmon, Atlantic (typically farmed)	Krill oil
Salmon, farmed	Salmon, Alaskan
Sea bass	Salmon, wild Pacific
Swordfish	Sardines
Tuna	Summer flounder
White croaker	

Conventional Yogurt

Yogurt is having its moment. Per capita yogurt consumption has doubled over the last decade, to the point that nearly one in three Americans now eats it regularly (according to a 2013 report by the market research firm NDP Group).[26] Greek yogurt in particular is experiencing a tsunami of popularity: in 2007 the strained, extra-creamy style of yogurt claimed only 1 percent of the yogurt market; by 2013 it had zoomed its way up to 35 percent, according to the *Wall Street Journal*.[27]

At first glance, yogurt seems a worthy recipient of our culinary devotion. It's a good source of protein, calcium, and probiotics, and it's easily packed in a lunchbox or stored in an office fridge.

Prepared in a traditional way—in which living cultures ferment raw milk from pasture-raised cows—yogurt *is* an excellent source of probiotics, saturated fat, vitamin D, calcium, and multiple beneficial enzymes. But when it's prepared as it is by the modern dairy industry, yogurt is reduced to a creamy junk food that provides little benefit beyond "mouthfeel"—the food industry term for how a food feels on the tongue.

The types of yogurt I'm talking about include any yogurt made with conventional dairy, whether it's low-fat, no-fat, flavored, plain, Greek, or regular. The primary problem with all conventional yogurt is that it is made with milk from cows raised on confined animal feedlot operations (CAFOs). These cows are denied access to their natural diet—grass—and instead are given corn and soybeans to eat. But the vast majority of corn and soybeans grown and fed to animals in the United States are genetically engineered. Moreover, corn is high in omega-6 fats, meaning that yogurt made from milk from corn-fed cows is also high in omega-6 fats.

Because cows evolved to eat grass, not corn and soy, their digestion is impaired. As you learned in Healing Principle 6, the gut makes up about 80 percent of immunity, so this diet switch makes cows more likely to get sick—as do their crowded living conditions, where they are often standing in a pool of their own manure. As a result, the cows are fed a host of antibiotics to keep them "well," if you can call it that, and producing milk. These antibiotics are then passed along in the milk to you.

Antibiotics aren't the only issue with cows fed grain instead of grass—milk from conventionally fed cows lacks nutrition. Organic milk has significantly higher levels of the antioxidants important for eye health—lutein and zeaxanthin—than does conventional milk.[28] Organic milk from pastured cows has also consistently been found to have higher levels of naturally occurring beta carotene (vitamin A) and tocopherols (vitamin E).[29] Milk from pastured cows is also a good source of omega-3 fats—a benefit that grain-fed milk doesn't share.

One substance administered to conventional dairy cows that is particularly troubling is recombinant bovine growth hormone (rBGH), a genetically engineered hormone designed to increase milk production. Numerous studies have found that milk from cows treated with rBGH has higher levels of insulin-like growth factor 1 (IGF-1).[30] When you drink milk or eat yogurt from rBGH cows, that IGF-1 makes it into your bloodstream, which is not a good thing: IGF-1 has been shown to increase the risk of breast cancer,[31] colon cancer,[32] and prostate cancer.[33] Not exactly a health promoter!

Another major issue with most conventional yogurts is that they are low-fat or no-fat. As I discussed just a few pages ago, saturated fat—the primary form of fat found in dairy—is an important part of a healthy diet. When some or all of the fat is stripped away, so is much of the nutrition offered by saturated fat. Saturated fats provide the building blocks for your cell membranes as well as a variety of hormones and hormonelike substances that are essential to health. When you eat fats as part of your meal, they slow down absorption so that you can go longer without feeling hungry. In addition, they act as carriers for important fat-soluble vitamins A, D, E, and K. Dietary fats are also needed for the conversion of carotene to vitamin A, for mineral absorption, and for a host of other biological processes.

Whole-milk dairy in particular is associated with important health benefits, including help with four of the most popular health problems in America today:

- **Diabetes.** Palmitoleic acid, which occurs naturally in full-fat dairy products, protects against insulin resistance and diabetes. One study found that people who consumed full-fat dairy had higher levels of trans-palmitoleate in their blood,[34] which translated to a two-thirds lower risk of developing type 2 diabetes compared with people with lower levels.

- **Cancer.** Conjugated linoleic acid (CLA), a type of fat found naturally in cow's milk, significantly lowers the risk of cancer. In one study, those who ate at least four servings of high-fat dairy foods each day had a 41 percent lower risk of bowel cancer than those who ate less than one.[35] Each increment of two servings of dairy products equaled a 13 percent reduction in a woman's colon cancer risk.
- **Weight.** Women who ate at least one serving of full-fat dairy a day gained 30 percent less weight over a nine-year period than women who ate only low-fat (or no) dairy products.[36]
- **Heart disease.** People who ate the most full-fat dairy were less likely to die from cardiovascular disease, according to a sixteen-year study of Australian adults.[37]

Another serious issue with reduced-fat dairy is the chemicals added to it, in part to give the creamy texture we've come to demand from yogurt. One such chemical is dimethylpolysiloxane, a chemical defoaming agent added to lowfat yogurt.[38] (It is banned from use in organic products.) Others are commercial thickeners and stabilizers, including carrageenan, xanthan gum, modified cornstarch, food starch, pectin and gelatin, artificial colors, and artificial flavors.

Carrageenan is particularly problematic, as it is known to trigger gastrointestinal symptoms, such as diarrhea and bloating.[39] It's heartbreaking to think of the folks who reach for yogurt and its probiotics because they are suffering from digestive issues, then making them even worse.

The other common additive to yogurt is perhaps the worst: sugar. Flavored yogurts can contain up to 27 grams of sugar per serving, making them as sweet, and often sweeter, than a candy bar. That's over six teaspoons of sugar in a single serving—more than four times the recommended daily intake. Even worse are the artificial sweeteners added to "light" yogurt products.

I rarely recommend eating pasteurized dairy products, as raw milk is such a superior form of nutrition. But if you, like so many Americans, have a yogurt habit, please—stick to plain, whole-milk, organic yogurt. If you prefer it sweeter, use stevia or lo han, or a teaspoon or two of raw local honey to sweeten it up.

Yogurt to Avoid	Better Choices
Low-fat yogurt	Organic plain whole-milk yogurt
Nonfat yogurt	Homemade yogurt made with organic, preferably grass-fed and raw, milk
Light yogurt	Homemade kefir (see recipe on page 168), made with organic, preferably grass-fed and raw, milk
Any yogurt made with nonorganic milk, including Greek yogurt	

Your Effortless Action Plan

1. As long as you have insulin or leptin resistance, drastically reduce or eliminate your grain intake.

2. Begin using stevia or lo han as your sweeteners of choice. Minimize your fructose consumption, and diligently avoid all artificial sweeteners—particularly aspartame.

3. Stop eating conventional soy and drinking soymilk. Eat only organic fermented soy.

4. Stick to organic virgin coconut oil for cooking and olive oil for salad dressings. Most other vegetable oils will harm your omega-6-to-omega-3 ratio.

5. Fish used to be universally healthy, but they're not anymore. Stick to summer flounder, wild Alaskan salmon, croaker, sardines, haddock, and tilapia, as they are least likely to be contaminated with mercury and other industrial toxins.

6. To ensure that you get enough omega-3 fats in your diet, consider taking a krill oil supplement.

7. Swap out any yogurt products you are currently eating with plain, organic, whole-milk yogurt. Even better, make your own yogurt or kefir with raw, pastured whole milk.

Part Three

Make It
Your Own

CHAPTER 3

Your Effortless Healing Plan

Healing Plan at a Glance

✿

✓ The key to creating lasting change is to set believable yet challenging goals.

✓ If you struggle to believe that you can meet your eating, living, and health goals, address your underlying emotional elements to truly embrace a new way of achieving those goals.

✓ Once you have the belief, the next thing you need is a plan.

✓ Tracking your progress with some quantifiable measurements will keep you motivated.

For some of you, implementing the recommendations of Effortless Healing will be easy, natural, and a nonissue. For the rest, it may take a little more time and diligence.

In this chapter, my aim is to help you use the information in this book to make lasting positive changes in your own life—and to do so in the simplest, easiest, and most efficient way possible.

Remember, living and healing are both a journey, not a destination. As you travel along your unique path, you will continue to fine-tune and optimize what works best for you and your life circumstances. If you are able to ease up on your program while maintaining optimal wellness—that is, if the seven factors listed on page 25 are all in a healthy range and you aren't experiencing troubling symptoms—then you are doing fine. But if any of your seven factors start to creep away from optimal ranges, your body is giving you feedback that you need to readjust. Just be honest with yourself.

What Comes First—Health or Happiness?

Your health and wellness play a significant role in your overall happiness. After all, it's tough to feel exuberant when you're not feeling well physically. Conversely, good mental health can bolster your physical health. As you start to clearly formulate your health goals, make sure to choose goals that will promote your long-term happiness. Instead of aiming to follow any advice to the letter, choose goals that will enable you to live more joyfully and effortlessly.

The Ten Components of an Attainable Goal

One of the best perspectives on goals that I know of comes from the book *Maximum Achievement* by Brian Tracy. To gain a greater understanding of the goal process and of creating the life you desire, I recommend that you review this book.

Making big changes is much more manageable—and possible—with a bit of forethought. Ten steps may sound like a lot, but the quantity of steps isn't what's important—it's the doableness of each step, and always knowing where you want to go and what you want to do next. Mapping out your goals will make them less overwhelming and much more empowering.

1. Identify the desire behind your goal.

Actions are usually based on either fear or desire. If you are fearful that you will remain sick always or will never achieve the weight or health you would like, then the odds are you are going to fail. Fear is a powerful force, yet it's not one that spurs us toward greatness. But desire is a burning that comes from within, and it has the power to change your very nature.

What exactly do you desire for yourself? Your answer must be entirely personal and must come from within. No one else can answer for you. It may take some digging, but once you answer the question, you activate your mind's innate goal-seeking mechanism. Once you have "programmed" a desire into your subconscious mind, your subconscious and your superconscious will take on a power of their own that will seem to drive and steer you to attain your goal, whatever it is.

2. Believe that achieving your goal is possible.

If you have any doubt in your mind about your ability to achieve something, you will unintentionally sabotage yourself. To achieve anything, you must fully and sincerely believe you can.

For a few of you, telling yourself that you are starting a new way of living and eating today and that you are going to follow it 100 percent may work. But you are the minority. You're far more likely to achieve your goals if you set a goal that you authentically believe you can achieve. This typically involves removing any emotional barriers and loving yourself even if you fail.

The goal you set must not only be one that you believe you can attain—it must also push you out of your comfort zone. That's where you must go if you want to create lasting change. It's a careful balance. To foster the belief in your ability to achieve a goal, stay focused on the short term—for instance, aim to eat grain-free for two weeks. You can adopt a new goal once you've gotten some success under your belt.

3. List the benefits you'll enjoy once your goal is attained.

The reasons you set your goal are the forces that will move you in the direction of attaining it. The reasons can be big or small. They may include having more energy, looking better, feeling great, walking your daughter down the aisle, living long enough to see your grandchild graduate, or fitting into a new dress. Whatever your personal reasons, write them down. Reviewing this list for a moment or two on a regular basis will help keep you motivated.

4. Write down your goal.

Having a goal—eating optimally, sleeping more, or getting a raise—is not a goal at all if it is not in writing. It is a fantasy, existing only in the ephemeral realm of your thoughts. Start an Effortless Healing journal, and begin by writing down your goal. Once you put your goal in writing, it will live outside your mind on the page. When your conscious mind can objectively see your goal—and not just catch fleeting glimpses of it when you remember to think about it—your goal will become more concrete.

Unfortunately, fewer than 3 percent of adults have clear

WRITE YOUR GOAL IN TWO WAYS

First, write down the details. Be specific—describe what your life will be like when you have met this goal. Let your imagination run wild. If your goal is to eat optimally, then write in detail what your meals will look like and what you will be able to do with all the energy you will have. Then place this description in an envelope to read when you need encouragement and motivation.

Second, write down your goal in one sentence, in the first person, and in the present tense. Your subconscious mind will respond only to commands that are personal, positive, and in the present tense. For instance, "I choose to eat only foods that add life and vitality to my organs and cells and to hydrate myself with clean, pure water." Write this sentence on several Post-it notes. Place them in your car, at your office, on your bathroom mirror, and by your bed.

Be careful to avoid using negatives. A little-known fact about the brain that is widely appreciated by those who practice energy psychology is that your mind will simply ignore the negative word before the goal and move you toward what you don't want. For example, if your goal is "I don't eat bread anymore," your mind will place the most weight on the word "bread" and essentially ignore the "don't." Ironically, you will command yourself to eat bread. A better goal would be "I effortlessly choose to snack on high-quality fats and vegetables."

Whatever goal you choose to write down, you want to be *very* clear about it. The three keys to achieving your goal are clarity, clarity, and clarity. Your success in life, and in Effortless Healing, will be largely determined by how clear you are about what you really want.

The more you write and rewrite your goal and the more you think about it, the clearer you will become about it. The clearer you are about it, the more likely you are to do more and more of the things that are consistent with achieving it.

written goals, with plans on how to achieve them. Typically, these 3 percent happen to be the people who are most successful in life at whatever they chose.

5. Recognize the obstacles.

Take a moment to think through anything that stands in the way of reaching your goal. The obstacles may be internal or external. An internal obstacle would be a certain belief about yourself or an attitude, such as: "I have too many things to do to get to sleep at a decent hour" and "People will think I'm weird if all of a sudden I start giving lots of hugs." An external obstacle is something outside of yourself, such as a spouse who brings you chocolate even though you're trying to stay away from it, or friends who like to eat out at Italian restaurants, when you're cutting down on carbs.

List all the obstacles you can think of. Then relist them in order of the difficulty of overcoming them.

6. Find support.

To achieve your goal, you are going to require help and encouragement from others. Your circle of support may include family, friends, coworkers, your doctor, and whomever else you deem appropriate. Be careful to select only those who you know will support and encourage you to the fullest.

Unfortunately, there are people out there who seem to sabotage others, especially when it comes to trying to lose weight or achieve better health. Educate the people you select about the reasons you are working toward your goal. If you present it well, they may even decide to join you—and then you will be really supported and held accountable!

7. Do a weekly review.

You will radically increase your chances of success if you review the progress you have made toward achieving your goal once a week. Do it when you are well rested, fresh, and relaxed. I implemented this habit over ten years ago, and it's become one of the most important practices I have. At the same time I also review my pending "action" items and "waiting for" folders in my e-mail.

8. Develop your plan for the next day or week.

Remember that if you fail to plan, you are planning to fail. So if healthy eating is your goal, then ideally you'd plan every meal for the upcoming week—say, on Friday before you go shopping—as this will radically increase your chances of success. If you can't plan for a whole week, at least plan for the upcoming day.

9. Visualizations

Visualizations are very powerful aids to achieving goals. Picture yourself sitting at a table and selecting only foods that add life and health to your body. Visualize participating in activities that provide energy. Picture how good you will feel when implementing the dietary recommendations. Imagine life with health.

The more detail you can add to your visualization, the more effective it will be. Take time each day to visualize. Do it at night before retiring, while rereading your written-down goal.

10. Make a commitment.

Surround yourself with those who support you and care enough about you to hold you accountable. We all have days, or weeks, where we slip. The important thing is that you realize it, admit it, and get back to taking care of yourself. As they said in *Apollo 13,* "Failure is not an option."

Addressing Your Emotional Roadblocks

M any people don't understand that emotional well-being is essential to their physical health. No matter how devoted you are to the proper diet and lifestyle, you will not achieve ideal health if emotional barriers stand in your way. In fact, if you have not been able to stay on a healthy living plan, emotional issues— whether it's a small ongoing anxiety or a serious trauma from the past—are likely a factor.

Maintaining negative thoughts and feelings about yourself can sabotage your efforts to take physical steps to improve your body. It will be like repeatedly washing your car during a dust storm. Fine-tuning your brain to "positive" mode is absolutely imperative for achieving optimal physical health.

To overcome emotional issues, you could choose a traditional psychological approach such as talk therapy. That can work, but there is a better solution. Psychological acupressure is an inexpensive, rapid, and proven way to eliminate the negative emotions that are barring you from a full and healthy life. And the EFT (Emotional Freedom Technique) is the most common form. If you feel that your emotions, or your self-image, may be your own worst enemy in following this (or any other) health and nutrition plan, I highly recommend you consider trying EFT. Please refer to page 213 for more information on this powerful method.

Regardless of how you do it, the most important step you can take to improve your health is stop *all* criticism of yourself. To make forward and lasting progress, you must stop criticizing yourself now and forever. Your thoughts create and contribute to all your experiences in life, especially as related to health issues. When you criticize yourself, you reinforce negative physiological changes. But when you approve of yourself, you facilitate positive changes throughout your life and your body.

If you have subconscious patterns that kick off a chain of inner criticism, you can change them. If you don't know how to stop thinking you are unworthy or undeserving, please, try EFT. It may seem "out there," but what have you got to lose, besides some very unkind thoughts?

If you don't love yourself when you are unhealthy, overweight, or struggling with debilitating symptoms, you are not likely to love yourself when you fit into skinny jeans or your blood pressure comes down. Trying to improve your health from a place of self-loathing will feel like punishment. But when you can come from a place of self-love, your efforts will feel effortless and your results more joyful. Self-acceptance is the crucial key to integrate into your life.

The good news is that you have a choice. You can choose to let go of the old pattern. You can choose to have different and more supportive thoughts. Letting go of your old negative pattern and replacing it with self-respect and love will allow you to move into a new pattern with ease. Please always avoid punishing yourself and beating yourself up.

Effortless Eating

The key to making dietary changes to achieve your goal is thinking ahead. If you wait to choose what you're going to eat until you're hungry, you're going to be tempted to reach for an old standby instead of make a new choice.

Every night before you go to bed, plan what you're going to eat the following day. Make the next day's lunch before you go to bed, because you typically have more time at night than in the morning before you go to work. Before you leave the house in the morning, determine what you will be eating for dinner. This will allow you to take the appropriate items out of the freezer or go to the store if necessary, rather than purchase unhealthy processed foods or go to a restaurant on the way home. If you don't plan in advance, you will likely slip back into your old, more comfortable, and less healthy eating habits.

Even better, make a weekly meal plan each weekend, and buy all the ingredients for that week's meals ahead of time so you're prepared. A big piece of carrying out a successful eating plan begins at the grocery store—you simply can't eat food that's not in the house.

Keep in mind that your eating plan doesn't have to be elaborate. You don't need intricately prepared dishes or three-course meals. You simply have to know what you'll be eating—it could be leftovers from the night before.

While variety is key, you really only need ten recipes that you know and enjoy. That may not seem like a lot, but that's all that most families use. Simply find those ten go-to recipes, and you will be paving the way for Effortless Healing. You might have to try ten to find one you really like, but view it as a game or a puzzle, and it will become fun and effortless.

If you are suffering from powerful cravings at any point, it is helpful to distinguish between physical food cravings and emotional food cravings. If you crave sweets or grains because of an emotional challenge, you will continue to battle that craving until you address the underlying emotions. I know, it may seem daunting to unpack the emotions you've been stuffing way, way down with food. But the very effective and simple techniques I've mentioned will make this type of work very doable. And the relief you'll feel will be palpable, freeing up enormous amounts of energy that you can then use toward making changes.

If you are hungry, frequently it is a symptom of dehydration. Simply drink a glass of pure water or tea and wait fifteen minutes. You will find that the hunger cravings often will disappear.

If you crave sweets because your body is used to burning sugar rather than fat for fuel—because up until this point you have been primarily feeding yourself grains and other unhealthy carbs—your best option for quelling the craving is to eat a good source of high-quality fat. A handful of olives or macadamia nuts, a green juice with a spoonful of coconut oil blended in it, or a glass of homemade whole-milk kefir with a few drops of stevia or lo han will take the edge off that sugar urge while helping your body make the transition to burning fat. Remember that these physiological cravings are short-lived: once you do start burning fat as your main form of fuel, the sugar cravings will typically disappear altogether.

It is also common for people to crave ingredients they are intolerant of or allergic to. If you struggle with a strong craving for a particular food, such as dairy or sugar, know that it will subside after your body has had a chance to heal from the sensitivity. Let the knowledge that eating that longed-for food will only perpetuate your subpar health steer you toward choosing a healthier option.

Effortless Health

At the beginning of this book, I counseled you to check the current status of your seven factors of health—fasting insulin level, vitamin D level, waist-to-hip ratio, body fat percentage, cholesterol and HDL ratios, blood pressure, and uric acid level. As you implement Effortless Healing, revisit the seven factors, as they are your best quantitative indicator of how the changes you're making are paying off. Whatever you focus on tends to grow. Seeing proof of success is motivating. So monitoring these seven factors will be an important step in improving your health.

Factor	Starting date	6 months from now	1 year from now
[Fasting] insulin level			
Vitamin D level			
Waist-to-hip ratio			
Body fat percentage			
Cholesterol and HDL ratios			
Blood pressure			
Uric acid level			

Other areas that are helpful to keep track of are sleep, hydration, and grounding activities—such as hugging, kissing, laughing, having sex, and walking barefoot (as discussed in Healing Principle 8). Every day, in the journal where you wrote down your goal or in your daily calendar, give yourself a score of 1 to 10 in each of these three areas, 1 being the lowest, meaning this area has gone completely off the rails, and 10 being the highest, meaning this area is absolutely great. If these numbers are holding steady at an 8 or above, you're doing well. If any are stuck at a suboptimal level or trending downward, ask yourself what it would take to get that number up a point or two; write down a new goal based on that reflection.

Category	Rating
Sleep	
Hydration	
Grounding	

Effortless Living

I n this book I've given you nine Healing Principles, nine ways to create the conditions for Effortless Healing in your own body. I've packed as much information as I can into these pages so that you'll be armed with the details on how to implement them. And yet even with all those suggestions, I want you to close this book with a clear vision of how to implement them in a way that feels effortless.

Remember, you don't have to start in all nine areas at once. Start small, and keep going. Each new habit you create will have a big effect on how you feel. The more days, weeks, and months you follow a new routine, the more energy and motivation you'll have to implement another change. You may not be ready to start performing high-intensity interval training today; but after a month of dramatically reducing or cutting out soda, for example, you'll be much more empowered and energetic than you are today and perhaps ready to add a new form of exercise.

To help with your visualization process, here's what a week's activities that promote Effortless Healing look like. My hope is that it will show you that the time commitment is minimal compared to the benefits you'll reap.

A Sample Week of Effortless Living

Monday

| MEAL |

Breakfast (optional): Vegetable juice with a teaspoon of coconut oil mixed in

Lunch: Large salad with mixed greens, sprouts, avocado, red peppers, fermented vegetables

Snack: ¼ cup of raw Macadamia nuts

Dinner: 1–2 braised pastured chicken thighs; raw tomatoes and cucumbers sprinkled with a little feta cheese, olive oil, and red wine vinegar

| ACTIVITY |

High-intensity interval workout, 20 minutes

Active isolated stretching, 10 minutes

Total duration: 30 minutes

Benefit: Increased human growth hormone and fat-burning enzymes

| ADVANCED EFFORTLESS HEALING |

Exercise outside with at least 40% of your skin exposed

Benefit: Vitamin D production

Tuesday

| MEAL |

Breakfast (optional): 1–2 pastured eggs, ideally raw or lightly cooked (soft-boiled or poached); sliced tomatoes; a glass of raw milk

Lunch: Large salad with sprouts, mushrooms, cucumbers, pecans, olive oil, and balsamic vinegar

Snack: Celery and cucumber dipped in a miso/tahini dressing

Dinner: 4- to 6-ounce organic grass-fed beef (burger or steak) and greens sautéed in pastured butter

| ACTIVITY |

Gardening, if seasonally appropriate

Total duration: 45 minutes

Benefit: Strength training, exposure to circadian-rhythm regulating sunlight

| ADVANCED EFFORTLESS HEALING |

Go barefoot for at least 20 minutes of your outside time

Benefit: Literal grounding and its anti-inflammatory and sleep-promoting effects

Wednesday

| MEAL |

Breakfast: Skip

Lunch: Leftovers from dinner the night before (be sure to make extra the night before if you choose this option)

Snack: Glass of kefir sweetened with stevia and ¼ teaspoon vanilla

Dinner: Stir-fry of 6 ounces ground beef or chicken with vegetables (if you are working on healing insulin and leptin resistance, substitute lightly steamed and diced cauliflower for rice)

| ACTIVITY |

Enjoy a stretching routine soon after you awaken. *Benefit:* Promotes relaxation, wards off aches and pains

Strength training, 20 minutes. *Benefit:* Increased human growth hormone and fat-burning enzymes

Total duration: 35 minutes

| ADVANCED EFFORTLESS HEALING |

Make it a screen-free digital detox night

Benefit: Encourages healthy melatonin production and thus sleep

Thursday

| MEAL |

Breakfast: Vegetable juice with a teaspoon of coconut oil mixed in

Lunch: Thai chicken soup, preferably made with homemade chicken stock, coconut milk, and lemon juice to taste

Snack: Olives and a couple of slices of raw milk cheese

Dinner: 1–2 grilled pastured drumsticks or thighs with homemade guacamole and a green salad with sprouts

| ACTIVITY |

High-intensity interval training workout, 20 minutes

Total duration: 40 minutes

Benefit: Increased human growth hormone and fat-burning enzymes

| ADVANCED EFFORTLESS HEALING |

Exercise first thing in the morning; if you choose to eat breakfast, delay it until after you've worked out

Benefit: Further boost to human growth hormone and fat-burning enzyme production

Friday

| MEAL |

Breakfast: Skip

Lunch: Leftover soup, large salad with fresh mixed greens, cucumbers, celery, mushrooms, olive oil, and balsamic vinegar

Snack: A handful of pecans

Dinner: 6–8 ounces wild Alaskan salmon with lemon and butter, tossed kale salad

| ACTIVITY |

Eat your lunch outside

Total duration: 20 minutes

Benefit: Exposure to circadian-rhythm regulating and mood-boosting sunlight

| ADVANCED EFFORTLESS HEALING |

Kick off your shoes and keep both feet on the ground as you eat and expose 40% or more of your skin

Benefit: Stress reduction, anti-inflammatory effects, and increased vitamin D

Saturday

| MEAL |

Breakfast: Skip

Lunch: Cream of broccoli soup, made with homemade chicken stock, broccoli, plenty of pastured butter, and enough raw, pastured cream to make it delectable

Snack: Celery and cucumber spears dipped in miso-tahini dressing; glass of fresh green juice

Dinner: 6-ounce grass-fed steak or ground buffalo burger, without the bun

| ACTIVITY |

Walk to farmers' market, buy pastured eggs and organic veggies

Total duration: 60 minutes

Benefit: Improved circulation, exposure to natural light, peace of mind that comes from buying the highest-possible-quality food (local, organic, and pastured)

| ADVANCED EFFORTLESS HEALING |

Make some fermented vegetables

Benefit: Improve your microbiome and obtain vitamin K_2 to balance your vitamin D levels

Sunday

| MEAL |

Breakfast: 1–2 pastured eggs, ideally raw or lightly cooked (soft-boiled or poached); sliced tomaoes; a glass of raw milk

Lunch: Leftover soup

Snack: Olives and a couple of slices of raw milk cheese

Dinner: A Sunday roast of grass-fed, pastured meat with a large salad that includes sprouts and fermented veggies

| ACTIVITY |

Plan your meals for the week and write out a shopping list

Total duration: 30 minutes

Benefit: Peace of mind, dramatically increased likelihood of meeting goal to eat more healthfully

| ADVANCED EFFORTLESS HEALING |

Plant a tray of soaked sunflower seeds

Benefit: Access to some of the most nutrient-dense food there is

A Final Pep Talk

You are holding a road map to health in your hands. Whenever your journey stalls, come back to these nine principles. Check in on how you are doing with them: Are you drinking enough pure water? Crowding out the processed foods, sugary treats, and grains by eating (or drinking) your vegetables and getting enough high-quality fats? Are you nourishing your gut with fermented foods?

Remember, your body is an exquisite, intelligent machine. It wants to exist in its natural state, which is health. And it will effortlessly move toward and maintain health so long as you don't consistently subject it to things that interfere with these ingrained mechanisms. When you eliminate the most troubling and pervasive culprits that I've outlined in this book, you create the conditions required to reverse nearly every chronic disease. You reset your body's natural homing mechanism, which is toward health.

The question to continually ask yourself as you make decisions about what to eat and drink and how to live your life is:

Do I want to degenerate or regenerate?

The answer is simple. The power is yours.

You really can take control of your health.

Your Effortless Action Plan

1. *Write out your health goal using clear, positive statements. Be sure to review it once a week when you are rested and can commit to meditating on it.*

2. *Make a plan for the week ahead, mapping out what you'll eat, what you need to buy at the grocery store, when you'll get outside, and when you'll exercise.*

3. *Remember to start small and add more activities as your energy levels and vitality rise.*

4. *Measure your seven health indexes, and revisit them at least annually so you can monitor your progress.*

HEALERS	HURTERS
✓ Self-acceptance	✗ Self-judgment
✓ Writing out a clear, well-defined goal	✗ Merely thinking about a goal, especially in a vague way
✓ Planning out a week's worth of meals and a corresponding grocery list	✗ Waiting until you're hungry to think about your next meal and eating processed or restaurant food
✓ Addressing emotional issues that are sabotaging your desire to change	✗ Ignoring the emotional issues that may have led to your unhealthy habits in the first place
✓ Objectively monitoring your progress	✗ Forgetting to track your efforts and results

TIME TAKEN, TIME SAVED

It typically takes ten minutes to write out your most important goal (allowing time for you to mull it over and compose a couple of drafts before you hit on the clearest phrasing). But those ten minutes make you exponentially more likely to meet that goal. And when your goal is health-related, achieving it can add years to your life and add dramatic quality of life to those years.

NOTES

Chapter 1: What Effortless Healing Is, and Why You Need It

1. T. Philipson et al., "An Analysis of Whether Higher Health Care Spending in the United States vs. Europe Is 'Worth It' in the Case of Cancer," *Health Affairs (Project Hope)* 31, 4 (April 2012): 667–75: DOI: 10.1377/hlthaff.2011.1298.
2. C. Glenn Begley and Lee M. Ellis, "Drug Development: Raise Standards for Preclinical Cancer Research," commentary published in *Nature* 483 (March 29, 2012): 531–33: DOI: 10.1038/483531a.
3. Rebecca Rifkin, "U.S. Obesity Rate Ticks Up to 27.1% in 2013," Gallup Well-Being, February 27, 2014, http://www.gallup.com/poll/167651/obesity-rate-ticks-2013.aspx.
4. "Life Expectancy of U.S. Children Cut Short by Obesity," Ronald McDonald Children's Hospital, January 12, 2011, http://www.loyola medicine.org/childrenshospital/newswire/news/life-expectancy-us -children-cut-short-obesity.
5. "Introduction to the Health Care Industry," Plunkett Research, Ltd., http://www.plunkettresearch.com/health-care-medical-market-research/ industry-trends.
6. "Diabetes," Centers for Disease Control and Prevention, http://www .cdc.gov/chronicdisease/resources/publications/AAG/ddt.htm.
7. *2011 Alzheimer's Disease Facts and Figures,* Alzheimer's Association, http://www.alz.org/downloads/Facts_Figures_2011.pdf.
8. *World Cancer Report 2014,* World Health Organization, http://apps .who.int/bookorders/anglais/detart1.jsp?codlan=1&codcol=80&cod cch=275; Tim Hume and Jen Christensen, "WHO: Imminent Global Cancer 'Disaster' Reflects Aging, Lifestyle Factors," *CNN Health,* February 4, 2014.
9. S. J. Arbes Jr., P. J. Gergen, and Elliott L. Zeldin, "Prevalences of Positive Skin Test Responses to 10 Common Allergens in the U.S. Population," *Journal of Allergy and Clinical Immunology* 116, no. 2 (August 2005): 377–83, PMID: 16083793.
10. Brian Krans, "With 70 Percent of Americans on Medication, Have We Become a Pill Culture?" *Healthline News,* June 21, 2013, http://www

.healthline.com/health-news/policy-seventy-percent-of-americans-take
-prescription-drugs-062113.

11. Medco Health Solutions, "New Survey Shows Seniors Struggle Under the Weight of Multiple Medication Use," *PR Newswire,* December 29 (no year), http://www.prnewswire.com/news-releases/new-survey-shows-seniors-struggle-under-the-weight-of-multiple-medication-use-80246652.html.

12. Michelle Andrews, "Pharmacists Expand Role to Help Educate and Coach Patients," *Kaiser Health News,* March 15, 2011, http://www.kaiserhealth news.org/Features/Insuring-Your-Health/Michelle-Andrews-on-Pharmacy -Outreach-and-Chronic-Health-Problems.aspx; "Retail Prescription Drugs Filled at Pharmacies (Annual per Capita by Age)," Kaiser Family Foundation, http://kff.org/other/state-indicator/retail-rx-drugs-by-age.

13. Qiuping Gu, Charles F. Dillon, and Vicki L. Burt, "Prescription Drug Use Continues to Increase: U.S. Prescription Drug Data for 2007–2008," Centers for Disease Control and Prevention, *NCHS Data Brief* no. 42, http://www.cdc.gov/nchs/data/databriefs/db42.htm.

14. Cynthia M. Boyd et al., "Clinical Practice Guidelines and Quality of Care for Older Patients with Multiple Comorbid Diseases: Implications for Pay for Performance," *Journal of the American Medical Association* 294, no. 6 (August 10, 2005): 716–24, DOI: 10.1001/ jama.294.6.716; Paula A. Rochon, "Drug Prescribing for Older Adults," *UpToDate,* November 6, 2013, http://www.uptodate.com/contents/ drug-prescribing-for-older-adults.

15. "Chronic Conditions Among Older Americans," American Association of Retired Persons, 2014, http://assets.aarp.org/rgcenter/health/beyond _50_hcr_conditions.pdf.

16. Oregon State University, "One in Five Older Americans Take Medications That Work Against Each Other," *Science Daily,* March 13, 2014, http://www.sciencedaily.com/releases/2014/03/140313154220.htm; S. J. Lorgunpai et al., "Potential Therapeutic Competition in Community-Living Older Adults in the U.S.: Use of Medications That May Adversely Affect a Coexisting Condition," *PLOS-ONE,* February 25, 2014, DOI: 10.1371/journal.pone.0089447.

17. *Drug Abuse Warning Network, 2011: National Estimates of Drug-Related Emergency Department Visits,* U.S. Substance Abuse and Mental Health Services Administration, HHS Publication no. (SMA) 13-4760, http://www.samhsa.gov/data/2k13/DAWN2k11ED/ DAWN2k11ED.htm#high9.

18. Donna L. Hoyert and Jianquan Xu, "Deaths: Preliminary Data for 2011," *National Vital Statistics Reports* 61, no. 6 (Oct. 10, 2012), http://www.cdc.gov/nchs/data/nvsr/nvsr61/nvsr61_06.pdf.

19. "FAERS Patient Outcomes by Year," U.S. Food and Drug Administration, June 30, 2013, UCM070461.

20. "To Err Is Human: Building a Safer Health System," Institute of Medicine, National Academy of Sciences, November 1999, http://www.iom.edu/~/media/Files/Report%20Files/1999/To-Err-is-Human/To%20Err%20is%20Human%201999%20%20report%20brief.pdf; Marshall Allen, "How Many Die from Medical Mistakes in U.S. Hospitals?" ProPublica, Sept. 19, 2013, http://www.propublica.org/article/how-many-die-from-medical-mistakes-in-us-hospitals.

21. *Adverse Events in Hospitals: National Incidence among Medicare Beneficiaries,* Office of Inspector General, November 2010, oei-06-09-00090.

22. John T. James, "A New, Evidence-Based Estimate of Patient Harms Associated with Hospital Care," *Journal of Patient Safety* 9, no. 3 (September 2013): 122–28, DOI: 10.1097/PTS.0b013e3182948a69.

23. "Rules, Technology Leave Drug Reps Out of Luck," *American Medical News,* July 9, 2012, http://www.amednews.com/article/20120709/profession/307099947/5/.

24. Duff Wilson, "Harvard Medical School in Ethics Quandary," *New York Times,* March 2, 2009.

25. Jeffrey Kluger, "Is Drug-Company Money Tainting Medical Education?" *Time,* March 6, 2009.

26. H. L. Zuckerbraun, H. Babich, and M. C. Sinensky, "Triclosan: Cytotoxicity, Modes of Action, and Induction of Apoptosis in Human Gingival Cells in Vitro," *European Journal of Oral Science* 106, no. 2, pt. 1 (April 1998): 628–36, PMID 9584909.

27. "Triclosan: What Consumers Should Know," U.S. Food and Drug Administration, April 2010, UCM206222.

28. E. Matthew Fiss, Krista L. Rule, and Peter J. Vikesland, "Formation of Chloroform and Other Chlorinated Byproducts by Chlorination of Triclosan-Containing Antibacterial Products," *Environmental Science and Technology* 41, no. 7 (2007): 2387–94, DOI: 10.1021/es062227l.

29. "Chloroform," U.S. Environmental Protection Agency, January 2000, http://www.epa.gov/ttnatw01/hlthef/chlorofo.html.

30. Michael Moss, "The Extraordinary Science of Addictive Junk Food," *New York Times,* February 20, 2013.

31. Nell Boeschenstein, "How the Food Industry Manipulates Taste Buds

with 'Salt Sugar Fat,'" NPR, February 26, 2013, http://www.npr.org/blogs/thesalt/2013/02/26/172969363/how-the-food-industry-manipulates-taste-buds-with-salt-sugar-fat.

32. Kimber L. Stanhope, J. M. Schwarz, and P. J. Havel, "Adverse Metabolic Effects of Dietary Fructose: Results from the Recent Epidemiological, Clinical, and Mechanistic Studies," *Current Opinion in Lipidology* 24, no. 3 (June 2013): 198–206, DOI: 10.1097/MOL.0b013e3283613bca; Heather Basciano, Lisa Federico, and Khosrow Adeli, "Fructose, Insulin Resistance, and Metabolic Dyslipidemia," *Nutrition and Metabolism* 2, no. 5 (2005), DOI: 10.1186/1743-7075-2-5; Kimber L. Stanhope et al., "Consuming Fructose-Sweetened, Not Glucose-Sweetened, Beverages Increases Visceral Adiposity and Lipids and Decreases Insulin Sensitivity in Overweight/Obese Humans," *Journal of Clinical Investigation* 119, no. 5 (May 1, 2009): 1322–34, DOI: 10.1172/JCI 37385.

33. Matthias B. Schulze et al., "Sugar-Sweetened Beverages, Weight Gain and Incidence of Type 2 Diabetes in Young and Middle-Aged Women," *Journal of the American Medical Association* 292, no. 8 (2004): 927–34, DOI: 10.1001/jama.292.8.927.

34. Sanjay Basu et al., "The Relationship of Sugar to Population-Level Diabetes Prevalence: An Econometric Analysis of Repeated Cross-Sectional Data," *PLOS ONE* 8, no. 2: e57873, DOI: 10.1371/journal.pone.0057873.

35. Stephen Seely, "Diet and Breast Cancer: The Possible Connection with Sugar Consumption," *Medical Hypothesis* 11, no. 3 (July 1983): 319–27, PII: 0306987783900956.

36. Daniel Blumenthal and Mark Gold, "Neurobiology of Food Addiction," *Journal of Clinical Nutrition and Metabolic Care* 13, no. 4 (July 2010): 359–65, DOI: 10.1097/MCO.0b013e32833ad4d4.

37. Lauriane Cantin et al., "Cocaine Is Low on the Value Ladder of Rats: Possible Evidence for Resilience to Addiction," *PLOS ONE* 5, no. 7 (2010), DOI: 10.1371/journal.pone.0011592.

CHAPTER 2: BEFORE YOU BEGIN

1. http://articles.mercola.com/sites/articles/archive/2014/01/27/gout-uric-acid.aspx; http://articles.mercola.com/sites/articles/archive/2010/06/19/richard-johnson-interview-may-18-2010.aspx.

2. G. Ogedegbe et al., "The Misdiagnosis of Hypertension: The Role of Patient Anxiety," *Archives of Internal Medicine* 168 (December 8, 2008): 2459–65: DOI: 10.1001/archinte.168.22.2459.

HEALING PRINCIPLE 1: DRINK PURE WATER

1. N. S. Stachenfeld et al., "Mechanism of Attenuated Thirst in Aging: Role of Central Volume Receptors," *American Journal of Physiology— Regulatory, Integrative and Comparative Physiology* 272 (January 1, 1997): R148–R157, http://ajpregu.physiology.org/content/272/1/R148; Nannette B. Hoffman, "Dehydration in the Elderly: Insidious and Manageable," *Geriatrics* 46, no. 6 (June 1991): 35–38, PMID: 2040458; Risa J. Lavizzo-Mourey, "Dehydration in the Elderly: A Short Review," *Journal of the National Medical Association* 79, no. 10 (October 1987): 1033–38, PMC2625510.

2. "Dehydration: Symptoms," Mayo Clinic, February 12, 2014, http:// www.mayoclinic.org/diseases-conditions/dehydration/basics/ symptoms/con-20030056.

3. "Tap Water Toxins: Is Your Water Trying to Kill You?" (video), Mercola.com, February 7, 2009, http://articles.mercola.com/sites/ articles/archive/2009/02/07/tap-water-toxins-is-your-water-trying -to-kill-you.aspx.

4. "Powerade ION4," Coca-Cola Great Britain, 2010, http://www.coca -cola.co.uk/brands/powerade.html.

5. C. Trocho, "Formaldehyde Derived from Dietary Aspartame Binds to Tisso Components in Vivo," *Life Sciences* 63, no. 5(1998): 337–49, PMID: 9714421.

6. S. N. Bleich et al., "Diet-Beverage Consumption and Caloric Intake Among US Adults, Overall and by Body Weight," *American Journal of Clinical Nutrition* 104, no. 3 (March 2014): 72–78, DOI: 10.2105/ AJPH.2013.301556.

7. "A Guide to Glycols," Dow Chemical Co., http://msdssearch.dow .com/PublishedLiteratureDOWCOM/dh_0047/0901b803800479d9 .pdf?filepath=propyleneglycol/pdfs/noreg/117-01682.pdf&fromPage =GetDoc.

8. "Propylene Glycol," Agency for Toxic Substances and Disease Registry, n.d., http://www.atsdr.cdc.gov/substances/toxsubstance.asp?toxid= 240#12.

9. "Addendum to the Toxicological Profile for Propylene Glycol," Agency for Toxic Substances and Disease Registry, December 2008, http://www.atsdr.cdc.gov/toxprofiles/propylene_glycol_addendum.pdf?id=1123&tid=240.

10. "Propylene Glycol," Environmental Working Group, n.d., http://www.ewg.org/skindeep/ingredient/705315/PROPYLENE_GLYCOL/#.

11. "CSPI Downgrades Splenda from 'Safe' to 'Caution,'" Center for Science in the Public Interest, June 12, 2013, http://www.cspinet.org/new/201306121.html.

12. Mohamed B. Abou-Donia et al., "Splenda Alters Gut Microflora and Increases Intestinal P-Glycoprotein and Cytochrome P-450 in Male Rats," *Journal of Toxicology and Environmental Health, Part A: Current Issues* 71, no. 21 (September 18, 2008): 1415–29, DOI: 10.1080/15287390802328630; Susan S. Schiffman and Kristina I. Rother, "Sucralose, A Synthetic Organochlorine Sweetener: Overview of Biological Issues," *Journal of Toxicology and Environmental Health, Part B: Critical Reviews* 16, no. 7 (November 12, 2013), DOI: 10.1080/10937404.2013.842523; M. Yanina Pepino et al., "Sucralose Affects Glycemic and Hormonal Responses to an Oral Glucose Load," *Diabetes Care,* April 30, 2013, DOI:10.2337/dc12-2221; "Ask the Doctor: Are Artificial Sweeteners a Good Alternative to Sugar?" *Harvard Health Letter,* December 2011; X. Qin, "What Made Canada Become a Country with the Highest Incidence of Inflammatory Bowel Disease: Could Sucralose Be the Culprit?" *Canadian Journal of Gastroenterology* 25, no. 9 (September 2011): 522, PMID: 21912763; G. H. Lord and P. M. Newberne, "Renal Mineralization: A Ubiquitous Lesion in Chronic Rat Studies," *Food and Chemical Toxicology* 28, no. 6 (June 1990): 449–55, PMID: 2210518; Y. F. Sasaki et al., "The Comet Assay with 8 Mouse Organs: Results with 39 Currently Used Food Additives," *Mutation Research* 519, nos. 1–2 (August 26, 2002): 103–19, PMID: 12160896; S. W. Mann et al., "A Combined Chronic Toxicity/Carcinogenicity Study of Sucralose in Sprague-Dawley Rats," *Food and Chemical Toxicology* 38, suppl. 2 (2000): S71–89, PMID: 10882819; R. M. Patel et al., "Popular Sweetener Sucralose as a Migraine Trigger," *Headache* 46, no. 8 (September 2006): 1303–4, PMID: 16942478; "Heart Palpitations, Accelerated Heartbeat, Elevated Blood Pressure, Atrial Fibrillation," Splendasickness.blogspot.com, March 2006, http://splendasickness.blogspot.com/2006/03/heart-palpitations-accelerated.html.

13. "Acesulfame K: What Are the Cons?" in Betty Kovacs, "Artificial Sweeteners," Medicine Net, March 20, 2014, http://www.onhealth.com/artificial_sweeteners/page10.htm; "Acesulfame Potassium," International Programme on Chemical Safety, n.d., http://www.inchem.org/documents/jecfa/jecmono/v16je02.htm.

14. Sarah Kobylewski and Michael Jacobson, "Food Dyes: A Rainbow of Risks," Center for Science in the Public Interest, n.d., http://cspinet.org/new/pdf/food-dyes-rainbow-of-risks.pdf; Bernard Weiss, "Synthetic Food Colors and Neurobehavioral Hazards: The View from Environmental Health Research," *Environmental Health Perspectives* 120, no. 1 (January 2012): 1–5, PMC3261946.

15. "Ethoxylated Sorbitan Esters. Polysorbate-60," Mohini Organics Pvt. Ltd., http://www.indiamart.com/mohini-organics/ethoxylated-sorbitan-esters.html; "Polysorbate-60," Environmental Working Group, http://www.ewg.org/skindeep/ingredient.php?ingred06=705139; Roderick E. Black et al., "Occurrence of 1,4-Dioxane in Cosmetic Raw Materials and Finished Cosmetic Products," *Journal of AOAC International* 84, no. 3 (May 2001): 666–670(5), http://www.ingentaconnect.com/content/aoac/jaoac/2001/00000084/00000003/art00006.

16. P. Bendig et al., "Brominated Vegetable Oil in Soft Drinks: An Underrated Source of Human Organobromine Intake," *Food Chemistry* 133, no. 3 (August 1, 2012): 678–82, PII: S0308814612000921; "Should I Be Worried that My Favorite Soda Contains Brominated Vegetable Oil? What Is It?" Mayo Clinic, http://www.mayoclinic.org/healthy-living/nutrition-and-healthy-eating/expert-answers/bvo/faq-20058236.

17. "Brominated Vegetable Oil (BVO)," Nutrition 411, n.d., http://www.nutrition411.com/education-materials/miscellaneous-topics/item/2306-brominated-vegetable-oil-bvo.

18. Olga Naidenko et al., "Bottled Water Contains Disinfection Byproducts, Fertilizer Residue, and Pain Medication," Environmental Working Group, October 15, 2008, http://www.ewg.org/research/bottled-water-quality-investigation.

19. "Abstracts of Selected Bisphenol A (BPA) Studies," Breast Cancer Fund, n.d., http://www.breastcancerfund.org/assets/pdfs/tips-fact-sheets/bpa-abstracts.pdf; "Bisphenol A (BPA)," National Institute of Environmental Health Sciences, n.d., https://www.niehs.nih.gov/health/topics/agents/sya-bpa.

20. "Disinfection By-Products and the Safe Water System," Centers for

Disease Control and Prevention, n.d., http://www.cdc.gov/safewater/
publications_pages/thm.pdf.

21. R. Slovak, "Tap Water Toxins: Is Your Water Trying to Kill You?"
(video), Mercola.com. February 7, 2009, http://articles.mercola.com/
sites/articles/archive/2009/02/07/tap-water-toxins-is-your-water
-trying-to-kill-you.aspx.

22. Mayan P. C. Kutty and S. Al-Jarrah, "Disinfection By-Products—
Present Status and Future Perspective in Sea Water Desalination,"
presentation to the IDA World Conference on Desalination and Water
Reuse, Washington, D.C., August 25–29, 1991, http://bit.ly/1tFKcQT;
X. Zhang et al., *Characterization and Comparison of Disinfection
By-Products of Four Major Disinfectants. Natural Organic Matter and
Disinfection By-Products,* August 15, 2000, chap. 19, pp. 299–314,
http://pubs.acs.org/doi/abs/10.1021/bk-2000-0761.ch019; "Water
Treatment Contaminants: Forgotten Toxins in American Water,"
Environmental Working Group, February 2013, http://static.ewg.org/
reports/2013/water_filters/2013_tap_water_report_final.pdf; *Our
Children at Risk: The Five Worst Environmental Threats to Their
Health,* Natural Resources Defense Council, n.d., chap. 7, http://www
.nrdc.org/health/kids/ocar/chap7.asp.

23. "Neurobehavioral Effects of Developmental Toxicity," *Lancet Neurology* 13, no. 3 (March 2014): 330–38, DOI: 10.1016/S1474-4422(13)
70278-3.

24. "Prevalence and Severity of Dental Fluorosis in the United States,
1999–2004," Centers for Disease Control and Prevention, November
2010, http://www.cdc.gov/nchs/data/databriefs/db53.htm.

25. "Statements from European Health, Water, and Environmental
Authorities on Water Fluoridation," Fluoride Action Network, 2007,
http://fluoridealert.org/content/europe-statements/.

26. "WHO: Tooth Decay Rates in Fluoridated vs. Non-Fluoridated
Countries," Fluoride Action Network, August 21, 2012, http://
fluoridealert.org/content/who-data/.

27. "Communities That Have Rejected Fluoridation Since 2010," Fluoride
Action Network, 2013, http://fluoridealert.org/content/communities
_2010.

28. Mark D. Macek et al., "Blood Lead Concentrations in Children and
Method of Water Fluoridation in the United States, 1988–1994,"
Environmental Health Perspectives 114, no. 1 (January 2006): 130–34,

DOI: 10.1289/ehp.8319; Mark D. Macek et al., "Water Fluoridation and Blood Lead Levels in U.S. Children," *Journal of Public Health Dentistry* 63, suppl. 1 (2003): S36, http://www.slweb.org/macek-2003 .html; R. Masters et al., "Association of Silicofluoride Treated Water with Elevated Blood Lead," *Neurotoxicology* 21, no. 6 (December 2000): 1091–99, PMID: 11233755; R. D. Masters and M. Coplan, "Water Treatment with Silicofluorides and Lead Toxicity," *International Journal of Environmental Studies* 56 (1999): 435–49, http:// www.slweb.org/IJES-silicofluorides.html; Jay Seaveya, "Water Fluoridation and Crime in America," *Fluoride* 38 (2005): 11–22; "Dartmouth Researcher Warns of Chemicals Added to Drinking Water," *Dartmouth News,* March 15, 2001, http://www.dartmouth.edu/~news/ releases/2001/mar01/flouride.html.

29. X. S. Li, J. L. Zhi, and R. O. Gao, "Effect of Fluoride Exposure on Intelligence in Children," *Fluoride* 28, no. 4 (1995): 189–92, http:// www.slweb.org/li1995.html; Y. Li et al., "Effect of Excessive Fluoride Intake on Mental Work Capacity of Children and a Preliminary Study of Its Mechanism" (in Chinese), *Hua Xi Yi Ke Da Xue Xue Bao* 25, no. 2 (June 1994): 188–91, PMID: 7528715; Y. Lu et al., "Effect of High-Fluoride Water on Intelligence of Children," *Fluoride* 33, no. 2 (May 2000): 74–78, http://www.slweb.org/lu2000.html; L. S. Qin and S. Y. Cui, "The Influence of Drinking Water Fluoride on Pupils' IQ, as Measured by Rui Wen Standards," *Chinese Journal of the Control of Endemic Diseases* 5 (1990): 203–4; G. Wang et al., "Research on Intelligence Quotient of 4–7-Year-Old Children in a District with a High Level of Fluoride," *Endemic Diseases Bulletin* 11 (1996): 60–62; S. Wang et al., "Investigation and Evaluation on Intelligence and Growth of Children in Endemic Fluorosis and Arsenism Areas," *Chinese Journal of Endemiology* 24 (2005): 179–82; Q. Xiang et al., "Effect of Fluoride in Drinking Water on Children's Intelligence," *Fluoride* 36, no. 2 (2003): 84–94, http://www.slweb.org/xiang-2003 .html; Y. Yang et al., "Effects of High Iodine and High Fluorine on Children's Intelligence and the Metabolism of Iodine and Fluorine," *Zhonqhua Liu Xing Bing Xue Za Zhi* 15, no. 5 (October 1994): 296–98, PMID: 7859263; L. B. Zhao et al., "Effect of High Fluoride Water Supply on Children's Intelligence," *Fluoride* 29, no. 4 (November 1996): 190–92, http://www.slweb.org/zhao1996.html; Anna L. Choi et al., "Developmental Fluoride Neurotoxicity: A Systematic Review

and Meta-Analysis," *Environmental Health Perspectives* 120, no. 10 (July 2012): 1362–68, http://ehp.niehs.nih.gov/wp-content/uploads/120/10/ehp.1104912.pdf; Philippe Grandjean, "Neurobehavioural Effects of Developmental Toxicity," *Lancet Neurology* 13, no. 3 (March 2014): 330–38, PIIS1474-4422.

30. P. Mullenix et al., "Neurotoxicity of Sodium Fluoride in Rats," *Neurotoxicology and Teratology* 17, no. 2 (March–April 1995): 169–77, PII: 089203629400070T; J. D. Sharma, Deepika Sohu, and Parul Jain, "Prevalence of Neurological Manifestations in a Human Population Exposed to Fluoride in Drinking Water," *Fluoride* 42, no. 2 (April–June 2009): 127–32, http://www.fluorideresearch.org/422/files/FJ2009_v42_n2_p127-132.pdf.

31. Bradford D. Gessner et al., "Acute Fluoride Poisoning from a Public Water System," *New England Journal of Medicine* 330 (January 13, 1994): 95–99, DOI: 10.1056/NEJM199401133300203.

32. Ibid.; W. Lynn Augenstein et al., "Fluoride Ingestion in Children: A Review of 87 Cases," *Pediatrics* 88, no. 5 (November 1, 1991): 907–12, http://pediatrics.aappublications.org/content/88/5/907. abstract; Jay D. Shulman and Linda M. Wells, "Acute Fluoride Toxicity from Ingesting Home-Use Dental Products in Children, Birth to 6 Years of Age," *Journal of Public Health Dentistry* 57, no. 3 (September 1997): 150–58, DOI: 10.1111/j.1752-7325.1997.tb02966.x.

33. P. Barton Duell and Charles H. Chestnut III, "Exacerbation of Rheumatoid Arthritis by Sodium Fluoride Treatment of Osteoporosis," *Journal of the American Medical Association Internal Medicine* 151, no. 4 (April 1991): 783–84, DOI: 10.1001/archinte.1991.004000 40121028; Serpil Savas et al., "Endemic Fluorosis in Turkish Patients: Relationships with Knee Osteoarthritis," *Rheumatology International* 21 (2001): 30–35, http://link.springer.com/article/10.1007/s002960100132#page-1.

34. Committee on Fluoride in Drinking Water, National Research Council, *Fluoride in Drinking Water: A Scientific Review of EPA's Standards* (Washington, D.C.: National Academies Press, 2006).

35. Fred Pearce, *When the Rivers Run Dry: Journeys into the Heart of the World's Water Crisis* (Toronto: Key Porter Books, 2006).

36. Shalu Chandna and Manish Bathla, "Oral Manifestations of Thyroid Disorders and Its Management," *Indian Journal of Endocrinology and Metabolism* 15, suppl. 2 (July 2011): S113–S116, PMC: 3169868.

37. Elise B. Bassin et al., "Age-Specific Fluoride Exposure in Drinking

Water and Osteosarcoma (United States)," *Cancer Causes Control* 17 (2006): 421–28, http://link.springer.com/article/10.1007/s10552-005 -0500-6#page-2; Elise B. Bassin, "Association Between Fluoride in Drinking Water During Growth and Development and the Incidence of Osteosarcoma for Children and Adolescents," DMS thesis, Harvard School of Dental Medicine, April 2001, http://www.yes4cleanwater .org/secret/WordVersionsNowPDF/ArticleFmMary4Website.pdf.

38. Gerard F. Judd, *Good Teeth Birth to Death: The Prescription for Perfect Teeth*, rev. ed., Rexresearch.com, January 9, 1997, pp. 53–54, http:// www.rexresearch.com/judd/goodteeth.pdf.

39. J. E. Butler, M. Satam, and J. Ekstrand, "Fluoride: An Adjuvant for Mucosal and Systemic Immunity," *Immunology Letters* 26, no. 3 (December 1990): 217–20, PII: 016524789090149K.

40. Committee on Fluoride in Drinking Water, *Fluoride in Drinking Water*.

41. Ibid.

42. J. L. Gomez-Ubric et al., "In Vitro Immune Modification of Poly-morphonuclear Leukocytes Adhesiveness by Sodium Fluoride," *European Journal of Clinical Investigation* 22 (1992): 659–61, DOI: 10.1111/j.1365-2362.1992.tb01426.x.

43. Committee on Fluoride in Drinking Water, *Fluoride in Drinking Water*.

44. Murakonda V. Narayana and Niloufer J. Chinoy, "Reversible Effects of Sodium Fluoride Ingestion on Spermatozoa of the Rat," *International Journal of Fertility and Menopausal Studies* 39, no. 6 (1994): 337–46, PMID: 7889087; Niloufer J. Chinoy and Murakonda V. Narayana, "In Vitro Fluoride Toxicity in Human Spermatozoa," *Reproductive Toxicology* 8, no. 2 (March–April 1994): 155–59, PII: 0890623894900221; various authors and references, "Reproductive Effects of Fluoride Is [sic] Linked to Lower Birth Rates, Sperm, and Testosterone," Fluori-dation.com, http://fluoridation.com/sperm.htm#Fluoride%20Toxicity %20In%20Human%20Spermatozoa; Deogracias Ortiz-Pérez et al., "Fluoride-Induced Disruption of Reproductive Hormones in Men," *Environmental Research* 93, no. 1 (September 2003): 20–30, PII: S0013935103000598.

45. Y. Li et al., "Association of Vascular Fluoride Uptake with Vascular Calcification and Coronary Artery Disease," *Nuclear Medicine Communications* 33, no. 1 (January 2012): 14–20, DOI: 10.1097/ MNM.0b013e32834c187e.

46. Committee on Fluoride in Drinking Water, *Fluoride in Drinking Water*.

47. Eugenio D. Beltrán-Aguilar, Laurie Barker, and Bruce A. Dye, "Prevalence and Severity of Dental Fluorosis in the United States, 1999–2004," *NCHS Data Brief* no. 53 (November 2010), http://www.cdc.gov/nchs/data/databriefs/db53.htm.

48. *Guidelines for Drinking-Water Quality,* vol. 2: *Health Criteria and Other Supporting Information,* 2nd ed., World Health Organization, 1996; "Aluminum in Drinking-water," addendum to volume 2, http://www.who.int/water_sanitation_health/dwq/chemicals/en/aluminium.pdf.

49. Allan H. Smith et al., "Cancer Risks from Arsenic in Drinking Water: Implications for Drinking Water Standards," in W. R. Chappell, C. O. Abernathy, and R. L. Calderon, eds., *Arsenic Exposure and Health Effects* (Elsevier Science, 1999), http://asrg.berkeley.edu/Index_files/Publications_PDF/99SmithCancerRiskAsDW.pdf.

50. *Our Children at Risk: The Five Worst Environmental Threats to Their Health,* Natural Resources Defense Council, n.d., chap. 7, http://www.nrdc.org/health/kids/ocar/chap7.asp. Hend Galal-Gorchev, "Disinfection of Drinking Water and By-Products of Health Concern," World Health Organization for the Pan American Health Organization, n.d., http://www.bvsde.paho.org/bvsair/e/repindex/repi55_56/disdrink/dis.html; "Toxic Showers and Baths," Citizens Concerned about Chloramine, n.d., http://www.chloramine.org/toxicshowersandbaths.htm; "Toxic Water in Showers and Baths," Water Quality and Water Toxicity, n.d., http://www.toxicwatersolution.com/Water-Quality-and-Water-Toxicity/Toxic-Water-in-Showers; Valérie Bougault et al., "Airway Remodeling and Inflammation in Competitive Swimmers Training in Indoor Chlorinated Swimming Pools," *Journal of Allergy and Clinical Immunology* 129, no. 2 (February 2012): 351–58, PII: S0091-6749(11)01797-0; I. Anderson, "Showers Pose a Risk to Health," *New Scientist,* September 18, 1986; Robert Slovak, "Quality Healthful Water Matters—Now Let's Find It," *Public Health Alert,* n.d., http://aguadebaja.com/files/RobertSlovakArticle.pdf.

51. Gerald Pollack, interview by author, "The Fourth Phase of Water: What You Don't Know About Water, and Really Should," Mercola.com, August 13, 2013, http://articles.mercola.com/sites/articles/archive/2013/08/18/exclusion-zone-water.aspx.

Healing Principle 2: Eat Your Veggies
(Four Effortless Ways to Eat More)

1. Qanhe Yang et al., "Sodium and Potassium Intake and Mortality
   Among U.S. Adults: Prospective Data from the Third National Health
   and Nutrition Examination Survey," *Archives of Internal Medicine* 171,
   no. 13 (July 11, 2001): 1183–91, PMID: 21747015.

2. S. Boyd Eaton and Melvin Konner, "Paleolithic Nutrition: A Consid-
   eration of Its Nature and Current Implications," *New England Journal
   of Medicine* 312 (1985): 283–89, DOI: 10.1056/NEJM198501313
   120505.

3. Yang et al., "Sodium and Potassium Intake."

4. Eden Tareke et al., "Analysis of Acrylamide, a Carcinogen Formed in
   Heated Foodstuffs," *Journal of Agricultural and Food Chemistry* 50,
   no. 17 (2002): 4998–5006, DOI: 10.1021/jf020302f.

5. D. E. Corpet et al., "Colonic Protein Fermentation and Promotion of
   Colon Carcinogenesis by Thermolyzed Casein," *Nutrition and Cancer*
   23, no. 3 (1995): 271–81, DOI: 10.1080/01635589509514381.

6. R. Wijk and E. P. A. Wijk, "An Introduction to Human Biophoton
   Emission," *Forschende Komplementärmedizin* 12, no. 2 (2005): 77–83,
   DOI: 10.1159/000083763; F.-A. Popp, K. H. Li, and Q. Gu, eds.,
   Recent Advances in Biophoton Research and Its Applications (Singa-
   pore: World Scientific, 1992); F.-A. Popp et al., "Physical Aspects of
   Biophotons," *Experientia* 44, no. 7 (July 15, 1988): 576–85, DOI:
   10.1007/BF01953305.

7. B. Fuhrman et al., "Ginger Extract Consumption Reduces Plasma
   Cholesterol, Inhibits LDL Oxidation and Attenuates Development
   of Atherosclerosis in Atherosclerotic, Apolipoprotein E-deficient
   Mice," *Journal of Nutrition* 130, no. 5 (May 2000): 1124–31, PMID:
   10801908; Reza Alizadeh-Navaei et al., "Investigation of the Effect
   of Ginger on the Lipid Levels: a Double Blind Controlled Clinical
   Trial," *Saudi Medical Journal* 29, no. 9 (2008): 1280–84,
   10Investigation20080539.

Healing Principle 3: Burn Fat for Fuel

1. Joseph Mercola, "The Hidden Reason You Get Flabby (Not Calories
   or Lack of Exercise)," Mercola.com, April 30, 2012, http://articles

.mercola.com/sites/articles/archive/2012/04/30/fructose-and-protein
-related-to-obesity.aspx.

2. Ryan K. Masters, "The Impact of Obesity on U.S. Mortality Levels:
The Importance of Age and Cohort Factors in Population Estimates,"
American Journal of Public Health 103, no. 10 (October 2013): 1895–
1901, DOI: 10.2105/AJPH.2013.301379.

3. Thomas Seyfried, *Cancer as a Metabolic Disease: On the Origin,
Management, and Prevention of Cancer* (Hoboken, N.J.: John Wiley &
Sons, 2012).

4. Andrew W. Brown, Michelle M. Bohan Brown, and David B. Allison,
"Belief Beyond the Evidence: Using the Proposed Effect of Breakfast
on Obesity to Show 2 Practices That Distort Scientific Evidence,"
American Journal of Clinical Nutrition 98, no. 5 (November 2013):
1298–1308, DOI: 10.3945/ajcn.113.064410.

5. B. D. Horne et al., "Usefulness of Routine Periodic Fasting to Lower
Risk of Coronary Artery Disease in Patients Undergoing Coronary
Angiography," *American Journal of Cardiology* 102, no. 7 (October 1,
2008): 814–19, DOI: 10.1016/j.amjcard.2008.05.021.

6. B. D. Horne et al., "Relation of Routine, Periodic Fasting to Risk
of Diabetes Mellitus, and Coronary Artery Disease in Patients
Undergoing Coronary Angiography," *American Journal of Cardiology*
109, no. 11 (June 1, 2012): 1558–62, DOI: 10.1016/j.amjcard.2012
.01.379.

7. Michelle Harvie et al., "Dietary Carbohydrate Restriction Enables
Weight Loss and Reduces Breast Cancer Risk Biomarkers," *Genesis,*
n.d., http://www.abstracts2view.com/sabcs11/viewp.php?nu=P3-09
-02; Krista A. Varady and Marc K. Hellerstein, "Alternate-day Fasting
and Chronic Disease Prevention: A Review of Human and Animal
Trials," *American Journal of Clinical Nutrition* 86, no. 1 (2007): 7–13,
http://ajcn.nutrition.org/content/86/1/7.short; Michelle N. Harvie
et al., "The Effects of Intermittent or Continuous Energy Restriction
on Weight Loss and Metabolic Disease Risk Markers: A Randomized
Trial in Young Overweight Women," *International Journal of Obesity* 35
(2011): 714–27, DOI: 10.1038/ijo.2010.171.

8. Mariana S. De Lorenzo et al., "Caloric Restriction Reduces Growth of
Mammary Tumors and Metastases," *Carcinogenesis* 32, no. 9 (Septem-
ber 2011): 1381–87, DOI: 10.1093/carcin/bgr107; M. Mendivil-Perez,
M. Jimenez-Del-Rio, and C. Velez-Pardo, "Glucose Starvation Induces
Apoptosis in a Model of Acute T Leukemia Dependent on Caspase-3

and Apoptosis-Inducing Factor: A Therapeutic Strategy," *Nutrition and Cancer* 65, no. 1 (January 2013): 99–109, DOI: 10.1080/01635581.2013.741751; Rainer J. Klement and Ulrike Kämmerer, "Is There a Role for Carbohydrate Restriction in the Treatment and Prevention of Cancer?" *Nutrition and Metabolism* 8 (2011): 75, DOI: 10.1186/1743-7075-8-75.

HEALING PRINCIPLE 4: EXERCISE LESS AND GAIN MORE BENEFITS

1. Hidde P. van der Ploeg et al., "Sitting Time and All-Cause Mortality Risk in 222, 497 Australian Adults," *Journal of the American Medical Association Internal Medicine* 172, no. 6 (2012): 494–500, DOI: 10 .1001/archinternmed.2011.2174; R. Seguin et al., "Sedentary Behavior and Mortality in Older Women: The Women's Health Initiative," *American Journal of Preventive Medicine* 46, no. 2 (February 2014): 122–35, DOI: 10.1016/j.amepre.2013.10.021.

2. M. L. Irwin et al., "Randomized Controlled Trial of Aerobic Exercise on Insulin and Insulin-like Growth Factors in Breast Cancer Survivors: The Yale Exercise and Survivorship Study," *Cancer Epidemiology, Biomarkers and Prevention* 18, no. 1 (January 2009): 306–13, DOI: 10.1158/1055-9965.EPI-08-0531; R. Ballard-Barbash et al., "Physical Activity, Biomarkers, and Disease Outcomes in Cancer Survivors: A Systematic Review," *Journal of the National Cancer Institute* 104, no. 11 (June 6, 2012): 815–40, DOI: 10.1093/jnci/ djs207; Nashwa Nabil Kamal and Merhan Mamdouh Ragy, "The Effects of Exercise on C-Reactive Protein, Insulin, Leptin and Some Cardiometabolic Risk Factors in Egyptian Children With or Without Metabolic Syndrome," *Diabetology and Metabolic Syndrome* 4 (2012): 27, DOI: 10.1186/1758-5996-4-27.

3. Quoted in Alexandra Sifferlin, "Yoga and the Mind: Can Yoga Reduce Symptoms of Psychiatric Disorders?" *Time,* January 28, 2013. See also Joseph Mercola, "Benefits of Yoga: What the Research Says About Its Use for Common Health Problems," Mercola.com, February 22, 2013, http://fitness.mercola.com/sites/fitness/archive/2013/02/22/ yoga-benefits.aspx#_edn5.

4. Joan Vernikos, *Sitting Kills, Moving Heals: How Simple Everyday Movement Will Prevent Pain, Illness, and Early Death* (Fresno, CA: Quill Driver Books, 2011); "Sitting and Standing at Work," Cornell

University Ergonomics Web, n.d., http://ergo.human.cornell.edu/
CUESitStand.html; D. W. Dunstan et al., "Prolonged Sitting: Is It a
Distinct Coronary Heart Disease Risk Factor?" *Current Opinion in
Cardiology* 26, no. 5 (September 2011): 412–19, DOI: 10.1097/
HCO.0b013e3283496605.

HEALING PRINCIPLE 5: ENJOY THE
SUN AND GET YOUR VITAMIN D

1. Amin Salehpour et al., "A 12-Week Double-Blind Randomized Clinical
   Trial of Vitamin D_3 Supplementation on Body Fat Mass in Healthy
   Overweight and Obese Women," *Nutrition Journal* 11, no. 78 (Septem-
   ber 22, 2012), PMC3514135.

2. N. C. Bozkurt et al., "The Relation of Serum 25-hydroxyvitamin-D
   Levels with Severity of Obstructive Sleep Apnea and Glucose Metabolism Abnormalities," *Endocrine* 41, no. 3 (June 2012): 518–25, DOI:
   10.1007/s12020-012-9595-1.

3. W. B. Grant, "Hypertension," Vitamin D Council, n.d., http://www
   .vitamindcouncil.org/health-conditions/hypertension.

4. Angela Boldo et al., "Should the Concentration of Vitamin D Be
   Measured in All Patients with Hypertension?" *Journal of Clinical
   Hypertension* 12, no. 3 (March 2010): 149–52, DOI: 10.1111/
   j.1751-7176.2009.00246.x.

5. J. L. Anderson et al., "Relation of Vitamin D Deficiency to Cardiovas-
   cular Risk Factors, Disease Status, and Incident Events in a General
   Healthcare Population," *American Journal of Cardiology* 106, no. 7
   (October 1, 2010): 963–68, DOI: 10.1016/j.amjcard.2010.05.027.

6. Ricardo Castro, Derek C. Angus, and Matt R. Rosengart, "The Effect
   of Light on Critical Illness," *Critical Care* 15, no. 218 (2011), DOI:
   10.1186/cc1000.

7. Tissa R. Hata et al., "A Randomized Controlled Double-Blind Investigation of the Effects of Vitamin D Dietary Supplementation in
   Subjects with Atopic Dermatitis," *Journal of the European Academy of
   Dermatology and Venereology* 28, no. 6 (June 2014): 781–89, DOI:
   10.1111/jdv.12176.

8. John Cannell, "Is Curcumin Mimicking Vitamin D?" Vitamin D
   Council, June 19, 2013, http://www.vitamindcouncil.org/blog/is
   -curcumin-mimicking-vitamin-d.

9. M. Amestejani et al., "Vitamin D Supplementation in the Treatment of Atopic Dermatitis: A Clinical Trial Study," *Journal of Drugs in Dermatology* 11, no. 3 (March 2012): 327–30, PMID: 22395583.

10. P. Caramaschi et al., "Very Low Levels of Vitamin D in Systemic Sclerosis Patients," *Clinical Rheumatology* 29, no. 12 (December 2010): 1419–25, PMID: 20454816; A. Vacca et al., "Vitamin D Levels and Potential Impact in Systemic Sclerosis," *Clinical and Experimental Rheumatology* 29, no. 6 (November–December 2011): 1024–31, PMID: 22011638.

11. Thomas J. Wang et al., "Vitamin D Deficiency and Risk of Cardiovascular Disease," *Circulation* 117 (2008): 503–11, DOI: 10.1161/CIRCULATIONAHA.107.706127.

12. "Leading Causes of Death," Centers for Disease Control and Prevention, National Center on Health Statistics, December 30, 2013, http://www.cdc.gov/nchs/fastats/lcod.htm.

13. K. Madden et al., "Vitamin D Deficiency in Critically Ill Children," *Pediatrics* 130, no. 3 (September 2012): 421–28; DOI: 10.1542/peds.2011-3328; C. Rippel et al., "Vitamin D Status in Critically Ill Children," *Intensive Care Medicine* 38, no. 12 (December 2012): 2055–62, DOI:10.1007/s00134-012-2718-6.

14. P. Lee et al., "Vitamin D Deficiency in Critically Ill Patients," *New England Journal of Medicine* 360, no. 18 (April 30, 2009): 1912–14, DOI: 10.1056/NEJMc0809996; O. Lucidarme et al., "Incidence and Risk Factors of Vitamin D Deficiency in Critically Ill Patients," *Intensive Care Medicine* 36, no. 9 (September 2010): 1609–11, DOI: 10.1007/s00134-010-1875-8.

15. E. Smit et al., "The Effect of Vitamin D and Frailty on Mortality Among Non-institutionalized US Older Adults," *European Journal of Clinical Nutrition* 66 (September 2012): 1024–28, DOI: 10.1038/ejcn.2012.67.

16. William B. Grant, "A Review of the Role of Solar Ultraviolet-B Irradiance and Vitamin D in Reducing Risk of Dental Caries," *Dermato-Endocrinology* 3, no. 3 (July–September 2011): 193–98, DOI: 10.4161/derm.3.3.15841; William B. Grant, "Ultraviolet-B and Vitamin D Reduce Risk of Dental Caries," Vitamin D Council, September 27, 2011, https://www.vitamindcouncil.org/blog/ultraviolet-b-and-vitamin-d-reduce-risk-of-dental-caries.

17. Joseph Mercola, "Sensible Sun Exposure Can Help Prevent Mela-

noma, Breast Cancer, and Hundreds of Other Health Problems," Mercola.com, July 1, 2013, http://articles.mercola.com/sites/articles/archive/2013/07/01/vitamin-d-benefits.aspx#_edn7.

18. Sam Shuster, "Is Sun Exposure a Major Cause of Melanoma? No," *British Medical Journal* 337 (2008), DOI: 10.1136/bmj.a764.

19. Joseph Rivers, "Is There More Than One Road to Melanoma?" *Lancet* 363, no. 9410 (February 28, 2004): 728–30, DOI: 10.1016/S0140 -6736(04)15649-3.

20. N. J. Levell et al., "Melanoma Epidemic: A Midsummer Night's Dream?" *British Journal of Dermatology* 161, no. 3 (September 2009): 630–34, DOI: 10.1111/j.1365-2133.2009.09299.x.

21. M. Berwick et al., "Sun Exposure and Mortality from Melanoma," *Journal of the National Cancer Institute* 97, no. 3 (February 2, 2005): 195–99, PMID: 15687362.

22. Guangming Liu et al., "Omega 3 but Not Omega 6 Fatty Acids Inhibit AP-1 Activity and Cell Transformation in JB6 Cells," *Proceedings of the National Academy of Sciences* 98, no. 13 (June 19, 2001): 7510–15, DOI: 10.1073/pnas.131195198.

23. M. G. Kimlin, "The Contributions of Solar Ultraviolet Radiation Exposure and Other Determinants to Serum 25-Hydroxyvitamin D Concentrations in Australian Adults: The AusD Study," *American Journal of Epidemiology* 179, no. 7 (April 1, 2014): 864–74, DOI: 10.1093/aje/kwt446.

24. "EWG's 2014 Guide to Sunscreens," http://www.ewg.org/2014 sunscreen; Mercola, "Sensible Sun Exposure."

25. C. Masterjohn, "Vitamin D Toxicity Redefined: Vitamin K and the Molecular Mechanism," *Medical Hypotheses* 68, no. 5 (December 2007): 1026–34, PMID: 17145139.

HEALING PRINCIPLE 6: LET YOUR GUT FLOURISH

1. K. Tillisch et al., "Consumption of Fermented Milk Product with Probiotic Modulates Brain Activity," *Gastroenterology* 144, no. 7 (June 2013): 1394–1401, DOI: 10.1053/j.gastro.2013.02.043.

2. J. A. Bravo et al., "Ingestion of Lactobacillus Strain Regulates Emotional Behavior and Central GABA Expression in a Mouse via the Vagus Nerve," *Proceedings of the National Academy of Sciences* 108, no. 38 (September 20, 2011): 16050–55, DOI: 10.1073/pnas.1102999108.

3. P. Bercik et al., "The Anxiolytic Effect of Bifidobacterium Longum NCC3011 Involves Vagal Pathways for Gut-Brain Communication," *Neurogastroenterology and Motility* 23, no. 12 (December 2011): 1132–39, DOI: 10.1111/j.1365-2982.2011.01796.x.

4. Mark Lyte, "Probiotics Function Mechanistically as Delivery Vehicles for Neuroactive Compounds: Microbial Endocrinology in the Design and Use of Probiotics," *BioEssays* 33, no. 8 (August 2011): 574–81, DOI: 10.1002/bies.201100024.

5. Hans Bisgaard, "Reduced Diversity of the Intestinal Microbiota During Infancy Is Associated with Increased Risk of Allergic Disease at School Age," *Journal of Allergy and Clinical Immunology* 128, no. 3 (September 2011): 646–52, DOI: 10.1016/j.jaci.2011.04.060.

6. Tammy E. Stoker, Emily K. Gibson, and Leah M. Zorrilla, "Triclosan Exposure Modulates Estrogen-Dependent Responses in the Female Wistar Rat," *Toxicological Sciences* 117, no. 1 (2010): 45–53, DOI: 10.1093/toxsci/kfq180.

7. Gennady Cherednichenko et al., "Triclosan Impairs Excitation-Contraction Coupling and Ca^{2+} Dynamics in Striated Muscle," *Proceedings of the National Academy of Sciences* 109, no. 35 (August 2012): 14158–63, DOI: 10.1073/pnas.1211314109.

8. "FDA Taking Closer Look at 'Antibiotic' Soap," U.S. Food and Drug Administration, n.d., http://www.fda.gov/forconsumers/consumer updates/ucm378393.htm.

9. Joseph Mercola, "Do Air Pollutants Play a Role in Bowel Disease?" Mercola.com, October 5, 2013, http://articles.mercola.com/sites/ articles/archive/2013/10/05/air-pollutants-bowel-disease.aspx#_edn2.

10. A. Finamore et al., "Intestinal and Peripheral Immune Response to MON810 Maize Ingestion in Weaning and Old Mice," *Journal of Agricultural and Food Chemistry* 56, no. 23 (December 10, 2008): 11533–39, DOI: 10.1021/jf802059w; A. Aris and S. Leblanc, "Maternal and Fetal Exposure to Pesticides Associated to Genetically Modified Foods in Eastern Townships of Quebec, Canada," *Reproductive Toxicology* 31, no. 4 (May 2011): 528–33, PMID: 21338670; "Genetically Modified Foods," American Academy of Environmental Medicine, 2014, http://www.aaemonline.org/gmopost.html; Jeffrey M. Smith, "Dangerous Toxins from Genetically Modified Plants Found in Women and Fetuses," Institute for Responsible Technology, 2014, http://action.responsibletech nology.org/o/6236/t/0/blastContent.jsp?email_blast_KEY=1165644.

11. Sayer Ji, "Roundup Herbicide Linked to Overgrowth of Deadly Bacteria," GreenMedInfo, December 15, 2012, http://www.greenmed info.com/blog/roundup-herbicide-linked-overgrowth-deadly-bacteria.

12. Joseph Mercola, "A One on One Interview with Dr. Don Huber," Mercola.com, video transcript, December 10, 2011, http://mercola. fileburst.com/PDF/ExpertInterviewTranscripts/InterviewDrHuber -Part1.pdf.

13. M. B. Azad et al., "Gut Microbiota of Healthy Canadian Infants: Profiles by Mode of Delivery and Infant Diet at 4 Months," *Canadian Medical Association Journal* 185, no. 5 (March 19, 2013): 385–94, DOI: 10.1503/cmaj.121189; n.a., "Delivery Decision Is Nothing to Sneeze At," *Nature Medicine* 14, no. 11 (November 2008), DOI: 10.1038/nm1108-1169b; C. R. Cardwell et al., "Caesarean Section Is Associated with an Increased Risk of Childhood-Onset Type 1 Diabetes Mellitus: A Meta-Analysis of Observational Studies," *Diabetologia* 51, no. 5 (May 2008): 726–35, http://link.springer.com/ article/10.1007%2Fs00125-008-0941-z; S. Thavagnanam et al., "A Meta-Analysis of the Association Between Caesarean Section and Childhood Asthma," *Clinical and Experimental Allergy* 38, no. 4 (April 2008): 629–33, DOI: 10.1111/j.1365-2222.2007.02780.x.

14. Kerstin Berer et al., "Letter: Commensal Microbiota and Myelin Auto-antigen Cooperate to Trigger Autoimmune Demyelination," *Nature* 479, no. 7374 (October 26, 2011): 538–41, DOI: 10.1038/nature10554; H. Wekerle, "Natural Intestinal Flora Involved in the Emergence of Multiple Sclerosis," Max-Planck-Gesellschaft, October 27, 2011, http://www.mpg.de/4620085/intestinal_flora_multiple_sclerosis.

15. F. C. Westfall, "Molecular Mimicry Revisited: Gut Bacteria and Multiple Sclerosis," Nubiome: Cutting Edge Multiple Sclerosis Research, 2006, http://nubiome.com/blog/cutting-edge-multiple -sclerosis-research.

16. Joseph Mercola, "The Forgotten Organ: Your Microbiota," Mercola .com, December 9, 2013, http://articles.mercola.com/sites/articles/ archive/2013/12/09/microbiota-forgotten-organ.aspx#_edn12.

17. Souhel Najjar et al., "Neuroinflammation and Psychiatric Illness," *Journal of Neuroinflammation* 10, no. 43 (2013), DOI: 10.1186/ 1742-2094-10-43.

18. Michael Berk et al., "So Depression Is an Inflammatory Disease, but Where Does the Inflammation Come From?" *BMC Medicine* 11, no. 200 (2013), DOI: 10.1186/1741-7015-11-200.

19. Elizabeth A. Grice et al., "A Diversity Profile of the Human Skin Micro-biota," *Genome Research,* May 23, 2008, DOI: 10.1101/gr.075549.107.

20. L. B. von Kobyletzki et al., "Eczema in Early Childhood Is Strongly Associated with the Development of Asthma and Rhinitis in a Prospective Cohort," *BMC Dermatology,* July 27, 2012, DOI: 10.1186/1471-5945-12-11.

21. Jiyoung Ahn et al., "Human Gut Microbiome and Risk of Colorectal Cancer," *Journal of the National Cancer Institute* 105, no. 24 (2013): 1850–51, DOI: 10.1093/jnci/djt300.

22. Eva Sirinathsinghji, "The Gut Microbiome and Cancer," Institute of Science in Society, February 26, 2014, http://www.i-sis.org.uk/The_Gut_Microbiome_and_Cancer.php.

23. "Without This, Vitamin D May Actually Encourage Heart Disease," Mercola.com, July 16, 2011, http://articles.mercola.com/sites/articles/archive/2011/07/16/fatsoluble-vitamin-shown-to-reduce-coronary-calcification.aspx.

24. "Raw Milk Questions and Answers," Centers for Disease Control and Prevention, n.d., http://www.cdc.gov/foodsafety/rawmilk/raw-milk-questions-and-answers.html; Pam Schoenfeld, "B6, the Underappreciated Vitamin," Weston A. Price Foundation, April 1, 2011, http://www.westonaprice.org/vitamins-and-minerals/vitamin-b6-the-under-appreciated-vitamin/.

HEALING PRINCIPLE 7: CLEAN YOUR BRAIN WITH SLEEP

1. "Alzheimer's Facts and Figures," Alzheimer's Association, n.d., https://www.alz.org/alzheimers_disease_facts_and_figures.asp#quickFacts.

2. M. Irwin et al., "Partial Night Sleep Deprivation Reduces Natural Killer and Cellular Immune Responses in Humans," *FASEB Journal* 10, no. 5 (April 1996): 643–53, PMID: 8621064.

3. F. Campos-Rodriguez et al., "Association Between Obstructive Sleep Apnea and Cancer Incidence in a Large Multicenter Spanish Cohort," *American Journal of Respiratory and Critical Care Medicine* 187, no. 1 (January 1, 2013): 99–105, DOI: 10.1164/rccm.201209-1671OC; F. J. Nieto et al., "Sleep-Disordered Breathing and Cancer Mortality: Results from the Wisconsin Sleep Cohort Study," *American Journal of Respiratory and Critical Care Medicine* 186, no. 2 (July 15, 2012): 190–94, DOI: 10.1164/rccm.201201-0130OC; Anahad O'Connor, "Sleep Apnea Tied to Increased Cancer Risk," *New York Times,* May 20, 2012.

4. Lulu Xie et al., "Sleep Drives Metabolite Clearance from the Adult Brain," *Science* 343, no. 6156 (October 18, 2013): 373–77, DOI: 10.1126/science.1241224.

5. Irwin et al., "Partial Night Sleep Deprivation."

6. H. R. Wright, L. C. Lack, and D. J. Kennaway, "Differential Effects of Light Wavelength in Phase Advancing the Melatonin Rhythm," *Journal of Pineal Research* 36, no. 2 (March 2004): 140–44, PMID: 14962066.

7. Joseph Mercola, "Tips for Resetting Your Internal Clock and Sleeping Better," Mercola.com, August 15, 2013, http://articles.mercola.com/sites/articles/archive/2013/08/15/nutrients-better-sleep.aspx#_edn8.

8. Y. Wang et al., "A Metabonomic Strategy for the Detection of the Metabolic Effects of Chamomile (Matricaria recutita L.) Ingestion," *Journal of Agricultural and Food Chemistry* 53, no. 2 (January 26, 2005): 191–96, PMID: 15656647.

9. R. J. Reiter, L. C. Manchester, and D. X. Tan, "Melatonin in Walnuts: Influence on Levels of Melatonin and Total Antioxidant Capacity of Blood," *Nutrition* 21, no. 9 (September 2005): 920–24, PMID: 15979282.

10. Joseph Mercola, "Helpful Tips for Sleeping Better This Summer," Mercola.com, June 27, 2013, http://articles.mercola.com/sites/articles/archive/2013/06/27/better-sleep-tips.aspx#_edn8.

HEALING PRINCIPLE 8: GO BAREFOOT— AND OTHER WAYS TO STAY GROUNDED

1. K. M. Grewen et al., "Warm Partner Contact Is Related to Lower Cardiovascular Reactivity," *Behavioral Medicine* 29, no. 3 (Fall 2003): 123–30, PMID: 15206831.

2. G. L. Kovács, Z. Sarnyai, and G. Szabó, "Oxytocin and Addiction: A Review," *Psychoneuroendocrinology* 23, no. 8 (November 1998): 945–62, PMID: 9924746.

3. Cort A. Pedersen et al., "Intranasal Oxytocin Blocks Alcohol Withdrawal in Human Subjects," *Alcoholism: Clinical and Experimental Research* 37, no. 3 (March 2013): 484–89, DOI: 10.1111/j.1530-0277.2012.01958.x.

4. Ibid.

5. Marek Jankowski et al., "Anti-Inflammatory Effect of Oxytocin in Rat

Myocardial Infarction," *Basic Research in Cardology* 105, no. 2 (March 2010): 205–18, http://link.springer.com/article/10.1007/s00395-009 -0076-5#page-1.

6. Courtney E. Detillion et al., "Social Facilitation of Wound Healing," *Psychoneuroendocrinology* 29, no. 8 (September 2004): 1004–11, PII: S0306453003001902.

7. R. Fullagar, "Kiss Me," *Nature Australia* 27 (2003): 74–75.

8. Kory Floyd et al., "Kissing in Marital and Cohabiting Relationship: Effects on Blood Lipids, Stress, and Relationship Satisfaction," *Western Journal of Communication* 73, no. 2 (2009), DOI: 10.1080/ 10570310902856071.

9. C. A. Hendrie and G. Brewer, "Kissing as an Evolutionary Adaptation to Protect against Human Cytomegalovirus-like Teratogenesis," *Medical Hypotheses* 74, no. 2 (February 2010): 222–24, DOI: 10.1016/j.mehy.2009.09.033.

10. H. Kimata, "Kissing Reduces Allergic Skin Wheal Responses and Plasma Neurotrophin Levels," *Physiology and Behavior* 80, nos. 2–3 (November 2003): 395–98, PMID: 14637240.

11. Kara Mayer Robinson, "10 Surprising Health Benefits of Sex," WebMD, 2014, http://www.webmd.com/sex-relationships/guide/ sex-and-health.

12. David M. Selva et al., "Monosaccharide-Induced Lipogenesis Regu- lates the Human Hepatic Sex Hormone-Binding Globulin Gene," *Journal of Clinical Investigation* 117, no. 12 (2007): 3979–87, DOI: 10.1172/jci32249.

13. Michael Miller and William F. Fry, "The Effect of Mirthful Laughter on the Human Cardiovascular System," *Medical Hypotheses* 73, no. 5 (November 2009): 636, DOI: 10.1016/j.mehy.2009.02.044.

14. Keiko Hayashi et al., "Laughter Lowered the Increase in Postprandial Blood Glucose," *Diabetes Care* 26, no. 5 (May 2003): 1651–52, DOI: 10.2337/diacare.26.5.1651.

15. H. Kimata, "Viewing a Humorous Film Decreases IgE Production by Seminal B Cells from Patients with Atopic Eczema," *Journal of Psycho- somatic Research* 66, no. 2 (Feb. 2009): 173–75, PMID: 19154860.

16. Christina M. Pulchaski et al., "Spirituality and Health: the Develop- ment of a Field," *Academic Medicine* 89, no. 1 (January 2014): 10–16, DOI: 10.1097/ACM.0000000000000083.

17. David H. Rosmarin et al., "A Test of Faith in God and Treatment: The

Relationship of Belief in God to Psychiatric Treatment Outcomes," *Journal of Affective Disorders* 146, no. 3 (April 25, 2013): 441–46, http://www.jad-journal.com/article/S0165-0327%2812%2900599-X/abstract.

18. W. J. Strawbridge et al., "Frequent Attendance at Religious Services and Mortality over 28 Years," *American Journal of Public Health* 87, no. 5 (June 1997): 957–61, PMID: 9224176; Ronna Casar Harris et al., "The Role of Religion in Heart-Transplant Recipients' Long-Term Health and Well-being," *Journal of Religion and Health* 34, no. 1 (March 1995): 17–32, DOI: 10.1007/bf02248635; B. Coruh et al., "Does Religious Activity Improve Health Outcomes? A Critical Review of the Recent Literature," *Explore: Journal of Science and Healing* 1, no. 3 (May 2005): 186–91, PMID: 16781528.

19. Joseph Mercola, "Helpful Tips for Sleeping Better This Summer," Mercola.com, June 27, 2013, http://articles.mercola.com/sites/articles/archive/2013/06/27/better-sleep-tips.aspx#_edn8.

20. Gaétan Chevalier et al., "Earthing: Health Implications of Reconnecting the Human Body to the Earth's Surface Electrons," *Journal of Environmental and Public Health* (2012), DOI: 10.1155/jeph/2012-291541.

21. Stephen Sinatra, "The Earthing Benefits for Heart Health," DrSinatra.com, February 22, 2014, http://www.drsinatra.com/the-earthing-benefits-for-heart-health.

22. T. J. Black, "Can I Tell If Concrete Sealant Was Applied?" eHow, n.d., http://www.ehow.com/way_5863574_can-tell-concrete-sealant-applied_.html.

23. Dawson Church, Garret Yount, and Audrey J. Brooks, "The Effect of Emotional Freedom Techniques on Stress Biochemistry: A Randomized Controlled Trial," *Journal of Nervous and Mental Disease* 200, no. 10 (October 2012): 891–96, DOI: 10.1097/NMD.0b013e31826b9fc1.

24. Dawson Church et al., "Psychological Trauma Symptom Improvement in Veterans Using Emotional Freedom Techniques: A Randomized Controlled Trial," *Journal of Nervous and Mental Disease* 201 (2013): 153–60, PMID: 23364126.

25. Dawson Church and Audrey J. Brooks, "CAM and Energy Psychology Techniques Remediate PTSD Symptoms in Veterans and Spouses," *Explore: Journal of Science and Healing* 10, no. 1 (2014): 24–33, DOI: 10.1016/j.explore.2013.10.006.

HEALING PRINCIPLE 9: AVOID THESE SIX "HEALTH FOODS"

1. D. C. Goff Jr., et al., "Insulin Resistance and Adiposity Influence Lipoprotein Size and Subclass Concentrations. Results from the Insulin Resistance Atherosclerosis Study," *Metabolism* 54, no. 2 (February 2005): 264–70, PMID: 15690322.

2. Tanja Stocks et al., "Blood Glucose and Risk of Incident and Fatal Cancer in the Metabolic Syndrome and Cancer Project (Me-Can): Analysis of Six Prospective Cohorts," *PLOS Medicine* 6, no. 12 (December 2009), DOI: 10.1371/journal.pmed.1000201.

3. A. Lindqvist, A. Baelemans, and C. Aerlanson-Albertsson, "Effects of Sucrose, Glucose, and Fructose on Peripheral and Central Appetite Signals," *Regulatory Peptides* 150, nos. 1–3 (October 9, 2008): 26–32, DOI: 10.1016/j.regpep.2008.06.008; K. L. Teff et al., "Dietary Fructose Reduces Circulating Insulin and Leptin, Attenuates Postprandial Suppression of Ghrelin, and Increases Triglycerides in Women," *Journal of Clinical Endocrinology and Metabolism* 89, no. 6 (June 2004): 2963–72, PMID: 15181085; Kathleen A. Page et al., "Effects of Fructose vs. Glucose on Regional Cerebral Blood Flow in Brain Regions Involved with Appetite and Reward Pathways," *Journal of the American Medical Association* 309, no. 1 (January 2, 2013): 63–70, DOI: 10.1001/jama.2012.116975.

4. C. Dees et al., "Dietary Estrogens Stimulate Human Breast Cells to Enter the Cell Cycle," *Environmental Health Perspectives* 105, suppl. 3 (April 1997): 633–36, PMID: 9168007; C. Y. Hsieh et al., "Estrogenic Effects of Genistein on the Growth of Estrogen Receptor–Positive Human Breast Cancer (MCF-7) Cells in Vitro and in Vivo," *Cancer Research* 58, no. 17 (September 1, 1998): 3833–38, PMID: 9731492.

5. L. K. Massey, R. G. Palmer, and H. T. Homer, "Oxalate Content of Soybean Seeds (Glycine max: Leguminosae), Soyfoods, and Other Edible Legumes," *Journal of Agriculture and Food Chemistry* 49, no. 9 (September 2001): 4262–66, PMID: 11559120.

6. E. Hogervorst et al., "High Tofu Intake Is Associated with Worse Memory in Elderly Indonesian Men and Women," *Dementia and Geriatric Cognitive Disorders* 26, no. 1 (2008): 50–57, DOI: 10.1159/000141484.

7. O. N. Donkor and N. P. Shah, "Production of Beta-Glucosidase and Hydrolysis of Isoflavone Phytoestrogens by Lactobacillus Acidophilus,

Bifidobacterium Lactis, and Lactobacillus Casei in Soymilk," *Journal of Food Science* 73, no. 1 (January 2008): M15–20, DOI: 10.1111/j .1750-3841.2007.00547.x.

8. Kee-Jong Hong, Chan-Ho Lee, and Sung Woo Kim, "Aspergillus Oryzae GB-107 Fermentation Improves Nutritional Quality of Food Soybeans and Feed Soybean Meals," *Journal of Medicinal Food* 7, no. 4 (Winter 2004): 430–35, DOI: 10.1089/jmf.2004.7.430.

9. Y. Tsukamoto et al., "Intake of Fermented Soybean (Natto) Increases Circulating Vitamin K_2 (Menaquinone-7) and Gamma-Carboxylated Osteocalcin Concentration in Normal Individuals," *Journal of Bone and Mineral Metabolism* 18, no. 4 (2000): 216–22, PMID: 10874601.

10. M. Kaneki, "[Protective Effects of Vitamin K Against Osteoporosis and Its Pleiotropic Actions]" (in Japanese), *Clinical Calcium* 16, no. 9 (September 2006): 1526–34, PMID: 16951479; D. Feskanich et al., "Vitamin K Intake and Hip Fractures in Women: A Prospective Study," *American Journal of Clinical Nutrition* 69, no. 1 (January 1999): 74–79, PMID: 9925126.

11. G. C. Gast et al., "A High Menaquinone Intake Reduces the Incidence of Coronary Heart Disease," *Nutrition, Metabolism and Cardiovascular Diseases* 19, no. 7 (September 2009): 504–10, DOI: 10.1016/j. numecd.2008.10.004.

12. N. Presse et al., "Low Vitamin K Intakes in Community-Dwelling Elders at an Early Stage of Alzheimer's Disease," *Journal of the American Dietetic Association* 108, no. 12 (December 2008): 2095–99, DOI: 10.1016/j.jada.2008.09.013.

13. K. Nimptsch, S. Rohrmann, and J. Linseisen, "Dietary Intake of Vitamin K and Risk of Prostate Cancer in the Heidelberg Cohort of the European Prospective Investigation into Cancer and Nutrition (EPIC-Heidelberg)," *American Journal of Clinical Nutrition* 87, no. 4 (April 2008): 985–92, PMID: 18400723.

14. K. Nimptsch, S. Rohrmann, R. Kaaks, and J. Linseisen, "Dietary Vitamin K Intake in Relation to Cancer Incidence and Mortality: Results from the Heidelberg Cohort of the European Prospective Investigation into Cancer and Nutrition (EPIC-Heidelberg)," *American Journal of Clinical Nutrition* 91, no. 5 (May 2010): 1348–58, DOI: 10.3945/ajcn.2009/28691.

15. D. W. Lamson and S. M. Plaza, "The Anticancer Effects of Vita-min K," *Alternative Medicine Review* 8, no. 3 (August 2003): 303–18, PMID: 12946240.

16. Penny M. Kris-Etherton, William S. Harris, and Lawrence J. Appel, "Fish Consumption, Fish Oil, Omega-3 Fatty Acids, and Cardiovascular Disease," *Circulation* 106 (2002): 2747–57, DOI: 10.1161/01 .cir.0000038493.65177.94.

17. T. M. Brasky et al., "Specialty Supplements and Breast Cancer Risk in the VITamins And Lifestyle (VITAL) Cohort," *Cancer Epidemiology, Biomarkers and Prevention* 19, no. 7 (July 2010): 1696–1708, PMID: 20615886.

18. H. Iso et al., "Intake of Fish and Omega-3 Fatty Acids and Risk of Stroke in Women," *Journal of the American Medical Association* 285, no. 3 (January 17, 2001): 304–12, PMID: 11176840; S. C. Larsson, N. Orsini, and A. Wolk, "Long-Chain Omega-3 Polyunsaturated Fatty Acids and Risk of Stroke: A Meta-Analysis," *European Journal of Epidemiology* 27, no. 12 (December 2012): 895–901, DOI: 10.1007/ s10654-012-9748-9.

19. M. Loef and H. Walach, "The Omega-6/Omega-3 Ratio and Dementia or Cognitive Decline: A Review on Human Studies and Biological Evidence," *Journal of Nutrition in Gerontological Geriatrics* 32, no. 1 (2013): 1–23, DOI: 10.1080/21551197.2012.752335; V. Solfrizzi et al., "Dietary Fatty Acids, Age-Related Cognitive Decline, and Mild Cognitive Impairment," *Journal of Nutrition Health and Aging* 12, no. 6 (June–July 2008): 382–86, PMID: 18548175.

20. Luisa Deutsch, "Evaluation of the Effect of Neptune Krill Oil on Chronic Inflammation and Arthritic Symptoms," *Journal of the American College of Nutrition* 26, no. 1 (February 2007): 39–48, PMID: 17353582.

21. A. P. Simopoulos, "Omega-3 Fatty Acids in Inflammation and Autoimmune Diseases," *Journal of the American College of Nutrition* 21, no. 6 (December 2002): 495–505, PMID: 12480795.

22. James J. DiNicolantonio, "The Cardiometabolic Consequences of Replacing Saturated Fats with Carbohydrates or Ω-6 Polyunsaturated Fats: Do the Dietary Guidelines Have It Wrong," *Open Heart* 1, no. 1 (2014): 1, DOI: 10.1136/openhrt-2013-000032.

23. Janet Larsen and J. Matthew Roney, "Farmed Fish Production Overtakes Beef," Earth Policy Institute, June 12, 2013, http://www.earth -policy.org/plan_b_updates/2013/update114.

24. Elsie M. Sunderland et al., "Mercury Sources, Distribution, and Bioavailability in the Ocean: Insights from Data and Models," *Global*

Biogeochemical Cycles 23, no. 2 (June 2009), DOI: 10.1029/2008GB003425.

25. "What You Need to Know About Mercury in Fish and Shellfish," U.S. Environmental Protection Agency, 2014, http://water.epa.gov/scitech/swguidance/fishshellfish/outreach/advice_index.cfm.

26. "Yogurt's Growth Primarily Sources to Young Adults and In-Home Breakfast, Reports NPD," January 29, 2013, https://www.npd.com/wps/portal/npd/us/news/press-releases/yogurts-growth-primarily-sources-to-young-adults-and-in-home-breakfast-reports-npd.

27. Sarah Nassauer, "The Greek Yogurt Culture War," *Wall Street Journal,* September 3, 2013.

28. T. Slots, J. Sorensen, and J. H. Nielsen, "Tocopherol, Carotenoids and Fatty Acid Composition in Organic and Conventional Milk," *Milchwissenschaft* 63 (2008): 352–55; Gillian Butler et al., "Fatty Acid and Fat-Soluble Antioxidant Concentrations in Milk from High- and Low-Input Conventional and Organic Systems: Seasonal Variation," *Journal of the Science of Food and Agriculture* 88 (2008): 1431–41, DOI: 10.1002/jsfa.3235.

29. Paolo Bergamo et al., "Fat-Soluble Vitamin Contents and Fatty Acid Composition in Organic and Conventional Italian Dairy Products," *Food Chemistry* 82, no. 4 (2003): 625–31, DOI: 10.1016/S0308-8146(03)00036-0; Slots, Sorensen, and Nielsen, "Tocopherol, Carotenoids and Fatty Acid Composition."

30. A. Daxenberger, B. H. Breier, and H. Sauerwein, "Increased Milk Levels of Insulin-like Growth Factor 1 (IGF-1) for the Identification of Bovine Somatotropin (bST) Treated Cows," *Analyst* 123, no. 12 (December 1998): 2429–35, PMID: 10435273.

31. Endogenous Hormones and Breast Cancer Collaborative Group, "Insulin-like Growth Factor 1 (IGF-1), IGF Binding Protein 3 (IGFBP3), and Breast Cancer Risk: Pooled Individual Data Analysis of 17 Prospective Studies," *Lancet Oncology* 11, no. 6 (June 2010): 530–43, DOI: 10.1016/S1470-2045(10)70095-4.

32. B. Jiang et al., "[Association of Insulin, Insulin-like Growth Factor and Insulin-like Growth Factor Binding Proteins with the Risk of Colorectal Cancer]" (in Chinese), *Zhonghua Wei Chang Wai Ke Za Zhi* 12, no. 3 (May 2009): 264–68, PMID: 19434535.

33. Alicja Wolk et al., "Insulin-like Growth Factor 1 and Prostate Cancer Risk: A Population-Based, Case-Control Study," *Journal of the National Cancer Institute* 90, no. 12 (1998): 911–15, DOI: 10.1093/jnci/90.12.911.

34. D. Mozaffarian et al., "Trans-palmitoleic Acid, Metabolic Risk Factors, and New-Onset Diabetes in U.S. Adults: A Cohort Study," *Annals of Internal Medicine* 1153, no. 12 (December 2, 2010): 790–99, PMID: 21173413.

35. Susanna C. Larsson, Leif Bergkvist, and Alicja Wolk, "High-fat Dairy Food and Conjugated Linoleic Acid Intakes in Relation to Colorectal Cancer Incidence in the Swedish Mammography Cohort," *American Journal of Clinical Nutrition* 82, no. 4 (October 2005): 894–900, PMID: 16210722.

36. Magdalena Rosell, Niclas N. Hakansson, and Alicja Wolk, "Association Between Dairy Food Consumption and Weight Change over 9 y in 19,352 Perimenopausal Women," *American Journal of Clinical Nutrition* 84, no. 6 (December 2006): 1481–88, http://ajcn.nutrition. org/content/84/6/1481.abstract.

37. M. Bonthuis et al., "Dairy Consumption and Patterns of Mortality of Australian Adults," *European Journal of Clinical Nutrition* 64 (June 2010): 569–77, DOI: 10.1038/ejcn.2010.45.

38. "M-I-03-14: Labeling and Standards of Identity Questions and Answers," U.S. Food and Drug Administration, October 3, 2003, http://www.fda.gov/Food/GuidanceRegulation/GuidanceDocuments RegulatoryInformation/Milk/ucm079113.htm.

39. "Carrageenan: How a 'Natural' Food Additive Is Making Us Sick," Cornucopia Institute, March 2013, http://www.cornucopia.org/ wp-content/uploads/2013/02/Carrageenan-Report1.pdf.

Acknowledgments

O n my first day of medical school I was given very clear instructions that most of what we learned in the next four years would be outdated by the time we graduated. I will always be grateful for that dose of reality provided by Dr. Ward Perrin, who believed the true purpose of school was to teach us how to be lifelong students of medicine. This advice fell on many deaf ears, but I found it to be one of the most powerful lessons from medical school. It has served me well my entire career.

Progress in any discipline is made on the shoulders of the giants that preceded us, and, with that in mind, I would like to acknowledge the tireless work of all the researchers who dedicated their lives to prevent the needless pain and suffering so many have had to endure.

Two recent individuals I greatly admire first come to mind: Dr. Fred Kummerow and Dr. Don Huber.

Dr. Kummerow, who is over a hundred years old, discovered more than seventy years ago the dangers of trans fats from processed vegetable oils. For decades he bravely fought an uphill battle providing clear research that saturated fats were not the enemy but rather the deadly recommendation to consume trans fats, which were gravely misguided. In 2013, his research led to a lawsuit that finally made the FDA acknowledge these fats could no longer remain on the Generally Recognized as Safe (GRAS) list. Junk food companies continue to fight this research, willing to sacrifice human lives for their bottom lines.

Dr. Don Huber is professor emeritus from Purdue and a retired colonel, serving forty-one years of active and reserve military service. He has fearlessly exposed the dangers of glyphosate and genetically engineered corn and soy, while being viciously attacked by the pesticide industry.

Nearly twenty years ago, Dr. Ron Rosedale played an integral role in my understanding of insulin and leptin resistance, and vastly increased my knowledge of their important connection to virtually all chronic disease. More recently, he mentored me in the practical application of nutritional ketosis, using high-quality healthy fats as a powerful tool to overcome this hormonal resistance.

I am also grateful to Ori Hofmekler for educating me about intermittent fasting. This information helped me integrate the right foods with the right time to eat. Krispin Sullivan is an innovative nutritional researcher who helped me understand the value of vitamin D and omega-3 fats more than a decade before they became popular in the media.

Dr. Natasha Campbell-McBride is a medical doctor in the UK. She practiced as a neurologist and a neurosurgeon for several years before starting a family. When her firstborn son was diagnosed with autism at the age of three, she was surprised to realize that her own profession had no answers. She developed the GAPS (Gut and Psychology Syndrome) program, which has taught me the enormous potential for and healing power of fermented foods.

A weeklong visit to the Hippocrates Institute in South Florida reignited my passion for growing sprouts, and led me to research how to produce nutrient-dense and inexpensive foods. I hope they will be grown in all households.

Dr. Ken Cooper first motivated me to start exercising nearly fifty years ago, but it wasn't until five years ago that Phil Campbell helped me refine my exercise habits. I've since incorporated high-intensity exercise as the basis of my workouts, which is a far superior alternative to conventional endurance workouts.

Dr. Joan Vernikos, a researcher with NASA for thirty years, has proven how dangerous sitting can be for individuals. The simple practice of standing up, stretching, and ensuring you never sit for too long at one time is crucial, as prolonged sitting *is an independent risk factor for chronic disease and early death—even if you exercise vigorously each week.*

Dr. Eric Goodman is a leading expert in posture and personally mentored me in how to sit and walk properly to help prevent long-term structural problems.

Clint Ober, an electrical engineer, introduced me to the concept of grounding, the process of allowing electrons from the earth to flow into our bodies to minimize inflammation, help structure the water in our body, and keep our blood flowing freely.

There are so many others I am very grateful to, including the 25,000 patients I treated during my twenty-five years in my clinic; they were important partners and friends as they pursued healthier, happier lives. There was nothing more rewarding than watching my patients improve their health, which motivated me to share this information freely on my website to the many millions who seek help.

I could have never reached so many people without the support of the hundreds of employees over the years who dedicated much of their time to helping me pursue my mission of changing the current health paradigm.

None of this would have been possible without my incredible parents and family: my dad, who instilled extraordinary self-discipline skills that in large part gave me the tenacity to endure; my mom, who lovingly nurtured, encouraged, and inspired me to pursue my passions; and my girlfriend, Erin, who has been a major support to me for the past five years.

INDEX

abdominal fat. *See* belly fat

acupuncture/acupressure, 212, 258

Aerobics (Cooper), 2

agave, 228–29, 231

age/aging
  and benefits of effortless eating,
    98
  dehydration and, 39, 40
  exercise and, 107, 117, 122, 125
  HGH and, 117
  insulin and, 25
  and resisting junk food, 237
  sleep and, 178
  sun and, 142
  thirst and, 40
  vitamin D and, 132

Agriculture Department, U.S.
    (USDA), 5, 68, 221, 235

allergies, 10, 150, 154, 159, 163, 196,
    198, 207, 225, 229, 233, 261

almonds, 101, 186, 191, 192, 226

Alzheimer's, 10, 22, 26, 28, 51, 97,
    118, 176, 180, 207, 236

American College of Gastroenterol-
    ogy, 171–72

American Council on Exercise, 28

*American Journal of Clinical Nutri-
    tion,* 43, 92

anaerobic exercise, 119, 120, 127

antibacterial soap, 155–56, 172, 173

antibiotics, 10, 155, 157–58, 171, 243

antioxidants, 78, 136, 141, 207, 241,
    243. *See also* uric acid

anxiety, 33, 152, 153, 161–62, 178,
    189, 213, 215, 233

Archives of Internal Medicine, 67

Arizona State University: kissing
    study at, 196

arsenic, 47, 51–52

arteries: hardening of, 131, 145

arthritis, 22, 50, 189, 196, 207, 236.
    See also osteoarthritis; rheuma-
    toid arthritis

artificial sweeteners, 41, 42, 43–45,
    164, 165, 227, 230, 232, 246, 247

aspartame, 43–44, 47, 227, 231, 247

assessment
  and beginning Effortless Healing,
    24–34
  recording of baseline, 34
  See also type of assessment

asthma, 10, 132, 159, 163, 189, 207

atherosclerosis, 30, 78, 130, 223,
    236

autism, 132, 159, 207

autoimmune diseases, 10, 17, 43, 158,
    159, 161, 164, 236

avocados, 64, 67, 70, 90, 100, 105,
    187, 191, 192, 239, 264

back pain: exercise for, 111, 123

barefoot, walking, 193, 194, 203–11,
    216, 217, 262, 265, 268

basal cell carcinoma (BCC), 134,
    136

bathing, 37, 38, 61. *See also* anti-
    bacterial soap; shower filters

Begley, Glenn, 9

behavior
  gut bacteria and, 158
  tracking, 190–91

belly fat, 19, 89, 97, 160

Benadryl, 189–90

blood pressure
  assessment of, 25, 32–33
  and benefits of sun, 130
  cause of high, 33
  dehydration and, 39
  effortless eating and, 95
  effortless health and, 261–62
  exercise and, 113
  fruit juices and, 75
  grounding and, 195, 211
  "health foods" and, 220, 221, 226
  ideal, 33
  insulin/leptin and, 89, 223
  laughter and, 198
  metabolic disorders and, 88
  pharmaceuticals for control of,
    32–33
  sleep and, 177, 178
  uric acid and, 33

ABOUT THE AUTHOR

DR. JOSEPH MERCOLA is a passionate advocate of natural medicine, a wellness champion, and a visionary who has implemented much-needed changes to our current health care system. For twenty-five years, Dr. Mercola treated thousands of patients at his wellness center near Chicago, and in 1997 he created Mercola.com, now the #1 natural health website in the world. A *New York Times* bestselling author, he has also appeared on national news media such as CNN, Fox News, ABC News, *Today,* CBS's *Washington Unplugged,* and *The Dr. Oz Show.*